The Management
of Traumatised
Anterior Teeth
of Children

The Authors

John Anthony Hargreaves

M.Ch.D. (University of Leeds), L.D.S. (University of Manchester).
Senior Lecturer in Operative Dental Surgery for Children and
Head of the Department of Children's Dentistry, University of Edinburgh.
Honorary Consultant in Children's Dentistry, South Eastern Regional
Hospital Board, Scotland.
Formerly Lecturer in Children's Dentistry, Universities of Leeds
and Manchester and Clinical Lecturer in Paedodontics at the Royal
Dental School, Malmö, Sweden.

John W. Craig

L.D.S. R.C.S. (Edinburgh), D.P.D. (University of St. Andrews).
Chief Dental Officer, City of Edinburgh.
Honorary Lecturer, Department of Preventive Dentistry, University
of Edinburgh.
Formerly Chief Dental Officer, County of Inverness, and Senior
Hospital Dental Officer and Honorary Clinical Lecturer,
Department of Children's Dentistry and Orthodontics, Dundee
Dental Hospital and School.

Foreword by
James Lorraine Trainer

L.R.C.P., L.R.C.S. (Edinburgh), L.R.F.P.S. (Glasgow),
L.D.S. R.C.S. (Edinburgh), F.S.A.
Chairman, Scottish Dental Estimates Board.

The Management of Traumatised Anterior Teeth of Children

John Anthony Hargreaves
John W. Craig

Foreword by
James Lorraine Trainer

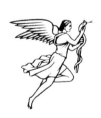

E. & S. LIVINGSTONE
EDINBURGH AND LONDON, 1970

ISBN   0   443   00621   0

Printed in Great Britain

Foreword

FEW emergencies in dental practice cause more distress than trauma to anterior teeth in children, particularly when those afflicted, as is so often the case, are patients who have been regular attenders anxious to maintain a sound dentition. Cases of this nature are much more common than is generally realised and it is disturbing to learn that the vast majority are untreated. Whether this is the result of inadequate knowledge or teaching in the past, it is difficult to estimate, but, despite the many advances in diagnosis and treatment which can help to alleviate these unfortunate occurrences, dental literature has given only sparse mention to the management of these patients.

This definitive work fills a long-felt gap and will do much to solve the problems with which practitioners are faced in the varying circumstances in which children's teeth are injured. Every likely calamity has been dealt with meticulously and thoroughly. After reading the book and becoming proficient with the proposed techniques, a dentist confronted with a damaged tooth in the young should be able to face his patient with complete confidence and equanimity. The chapters on radiographs as an aid to diagnosis, and the construction of basket and reverse retention crowns in intermediate treatment for injured incisor teeth, are particularly enlightening and worthy of careful study.

Treatment for children under 21 is available in Britain without charge on the National Health Service and every technique mentioned in this book is available to the general practitioner in the Service, with the exception of mouth protectors. With dental health education improving over the years and the recent intensive Government campaign to encourage the younger patient to attend regularly, it is hoped that many more will now avail themselves of the treatment procurable. This book will certainly assist the dentist to provide it.

The two authors, who combine academic teaching and practical knowledge in Hospitals and Local Authority clinics, have a vast experience in work of this nature and are an ideal combination. The text is well written and easy to read and assimilate. I consider the book to be required reading for all who are interested in paedodontics, whether students or graduates. It describes methods of treatment from which many young patients are likely to benefit and which all dentists will welcome.

I am glad of this opportunity of recommending a very valuable contribution to dental literature.

1970   J. L. TRAINER

Preface

THE growing interest in all aspects of dentistry for children has resulted in improved teaching of this subject at many dental schools throughout the world. As a result of this new awareness of child dental problems, the management of injuries to children's anterior teeth is now being taught to the undergraduate in a more systematic and comprehensive way. The dental student today has the opportunity to undertake the treatment of traumatised anterior teeth in a manner not available to his predecessor who, from necessity, has had to acquire his knowledge and skill in practice. Since the Second World War, dentistry has made rapid steps forward resulting in the development of more sophisticated techniques and the patient, rightly, has come to demand and expect more advanced treatment. Understandably there exists a variable standard of care, all too frequently falling short of the best that can be achieved. Many children in the past continued throughout childhood with untreated fractured incisor teeth or with functionally unsatisfactory restorations, often of poor appearance.

The purpose of this book is essentially to provide a companion to undergraduate teaching, but also to present in a clear and practical way a ready reference for the many dental practitioners and school dental officers who weekly have to face this problem, but who may not have had the opportunity of either undergraduate or postgraduate training in dealing with these unfortunate children.

A new and simplified classification of injuries to anterior teeth is set forth in the hope that it may provide an acceptable and readily understood form of common reference.

The subject is introduced by studying damage to the supporting structures of the tooth arising from both direct and indirect trauma, since it is considered that this approach provides a better basis for a thorough understanding of the injury as a whole.

Emergency and intermediate treatment is discussed in detail

for each type of injury and the text is so arranged as to provide a logical and systematic approach to treatment planning, but no attempt has been made, beyond the more important preliminary considerations, to discuss the preparation and construction of the final restoration. A brief chapter on the subject of prevention of injury has been included since we believe that susceptible children at risk should be protected wherever possible. Finally, the relevant laboratory techniques are set out in the Appendices.

In compiling this book we have consulted much of the current dental literature on the subject and although no author is quoted verbatim, we should like to record our appreciation to those colleagues whose publications have influenced our writing.

We are particularly indebted to Mr A. R. Bradshaw, Lecturer in Oral Medicine, Edinburgh University School of Dental Surgery, for the chapter on Radiographs as an Aid to Diagnosis and to Mr J. S. Clyde, Senior Lecturer in Operative Dental Surgery, Edinburgh University School of Dental Surgery, for the chapter on Pulp Therapy in the Traumatised Tooth. To both colleagues we wish to record our gratitude for their contributions. The laboratory techniques in the Appendices have been compiled by Mr J. Gray, Dental Instructor, Edinburgh University School of Dental Surgery, to whom thanks are also due.

In addition to the contributors we extend our thanks to Dr G. B. Hopkin and Dr C. E. Chapman who kindly read and criticised parts of the manuscript and to Mr D. M. McGibbon, who developed the method for bleaching teeth at Edinburgh Dental Hospital, for reading and criticising the technique described. The important task of reading the proofs was undertaken by Mr G. Bolas and for this, and his painstaking work in compiling the index, we should.like to express our warm appreciation.

The line drawings are the work of Miss Jenny Mitchell and Miss Mary Benstead, while the photographic illustrations were prepared by Mr Robert Renton, to all of whom we tender our grateful thanks for their artistic skill and accuracy. Our thanks are due to the editor and publishers of *Dental News* for permission to reproduce the illustrations on pages 50 to 53 and 87.

We acknowledge the willing help given by Miss Caroline

Graham, Miss Catherine Thomson, Miss Carolyn Lammiman and Miss Kathryn McWilliam in the typing of the manuscripts.

Finally, it is a pleasure to acknowledge the kindness and help we have received from the publishers at every stage in the production of this book.

J. A. H.

1970   J. W. C.

Contents

CHAPTER 1

The Problem, Prevalence, Aetiology and Classification

TRAUMA to the teeth of both permanent and deciduous dentitions is a very real problem met by all dental practitioners who deal with children. The treatment of injuries should always be commenced as early as possible following the accident. For this reason the initial treatment should be simple and rapid, so that a busy practitioner or school dental officer can deal with the emergency in his practice without having to delay drastically his daily appointments; it is of utmost importance that a quick method is used to arrive at an immediate and accurate diagnosis.

During childhood the development of the occlusion both functionally and aesthetically is dependent on the satisfactory presence of teeth. Unfortunate and disastrous results can occur when a traumatised region is inadequately treated, causing such conditions as malformed or malpositioned teeth, premature tooth loss and pulpal death with abscess formation (Figs 1 and 2).

The incidence of injuries to the anterior teeth among children at any particular age has been reported by several workers. Ellis (1960), who completed a survey of 4,251 secondary school children in Canada found that 4·2 per cent of these children had fractured anterior teeth and that fractures were two and a half times more common in boys than in girls. Further analysis of Ellis's figures showed that 73 per cent of the fractured teeth were upper central incisors, 18 per cent lower central incisors, 3 per cent upper laterals and 6 per cent lower laterals.

A similar survey undertaken by Craig in Edinburgh during 1966-67 found of 17,831 children examined between the ages of 4 and 18 years, 5·9 per cent had traumatised anterior teeth. Treatment of these injured teeth was minimal; 8·1 per cent had received satisfactory treatment, 2·8 per cent had received treatment considered unsatisfactory and 88·6 per cent had received no treatment.

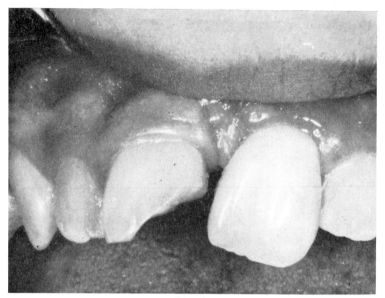

FIG. 1

Mesial drift and tilting of maxillary central incisors, following fracture of the right incisor which received no treatment.

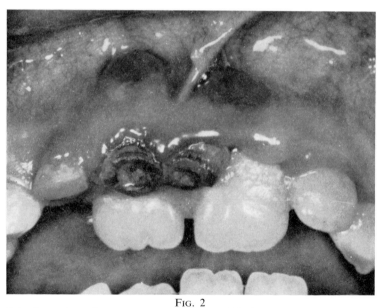

FIG. 2

Palatal eruption of permanent maxillary central incisors in a 7-year-old child following injury to the deciduous central incisors at 2 years of age. Development of apical abscess and failure of normal root resorption.

These figures show an increase in the incidence of fractured teeth compared with those given by Ellis, and this supports the view of other observers (Sweet, 1942; Zander and Law, 1942) who noticed even 25 years ago that the incidence of trauma to anterior teeth was increasing. This may be due to the more extensive gymnastic and sporting facilities available in both junior and secondary schools today, although other causes such as fights, accidental falls and, increasingly, car accidents play an important part in the cause of these injuries.

There is no doubt that boys suffer more injuries than girls even in the pre-school ages (Registrar General Reports, 1960; Hardwick and Newman, 1954). Accident proneness must also be considered and preliminary studies (W.H.O., 1957) suggest that children who are careless and come from broken homes are more prone to accidents than others. It is thought that this could be the result of emotional disturbances shown through physical behaviour.

In both the deciduous and permanent dentitions, several observers (Horsnell, 1952; Hallett, 1953) have shown that children with protruding teeth are more subject to fracture of their anterior teeth, and Brauer (1964) suggests that lack of adequate lip coverage may also be a contributory factor. Hallett found, in a study of 1,000 children, that the most common age of tooth trauma is between 8 and 11 years and children with maxillary protrusion—Angle Class II, division 1 malocclusion—are five times more susceptible to injuries of their anterior teeth than children with normal occlusion. Trauma to the deciduous anterior teeth was reported by Schreiber (1959), who observed 118 children who attended the Children's Department at Manchester Dental Hospital. He found deciduous anterior teeth were most commonly traumatised between 1 and 2 years of age, when children started to toddle and were still unsure of walking and running. Although many of the results of injury to the permanent and deciduous teeth are the same, the problems and consequences of trauma to the deciduous dentition are discussed in detail later.

IMMEDIATE RESULTS OF TRAUMA

A blow to the face may not cause permanent damage but can result in displacement, fracture, or both displacement and

TABLE I

Injury

	Displacement		Tooth Fracture
	Partial Displacement	Total Displacement	

Partial Displacement

By Direct Trauma
1 Palatal or lingual movement with fracture of the palatal or lingual alveolar bone.
2 Palatal or lingual movement with fracture of the labial alveolar bone and compression of the palatal or lingual alveolar bone.
3 Displacement of the tooth from its socket.

Total Displacement

By Indirect Trauma
1 Labial movement with fracture of the palatal or lingual alveolar bone and compression of the labial alveolar bone.
2 Labial movement with fracture of the labial alveolar bone.
3 Intrusion of the tooth into its socket compressing bone in the periapical region.

Tooth Fracture

1 Enamel fracture, not involving dentine.
2 Enamel and dentine fracture but no pulpal exposure.
3 Extensive crown fracture exposing the pulp.
4 Fracture of the root with or without coronal fracture.

fracture of teeth, with or without damage to the supporting and surrounding tissues (Table I). The direction and force of the blow can cause either direct or indirect injury to the teeth. Direct trauma occurs when a tooth is hit directly by an object such as a stone of hockey ball. Indirect trauma occurs when the mandibular teeth are forcibly closed against the maxillary teeth, usually as a result of a blow on the chin.

If the teeth are partially displaced, one of several conditions can occur.

Partial Displacement by Direct Trauma

In this case the teeth are usually displaced towards the tongue or palate and will appear either elongated or retroclined compared with the unaffected teeth.

The teeth displaced are generally maxillary central incisors of a young child where the roots are incompletely formed and the cancellous bone of the maxilla is less dense than in the adult. The tooth, therefore, with less support against a sudden blow, displaces with relative ease.

The displacement normally follows one of three movements:

1. A palatal or lingual movement with fracture of the palatal or lingual alveolar bone (Fig. 3A).
2. A palatal or lingual movement with fracture of the labial alveolar bone and compression of the palatal or lingual alveolar bone (Fig. 3B).
3. Displacement of the tooth from its socket, the tooth appearing elongated on clinical examination (Fig. 3C).

Partial Displacement by Indirect Trauma

Indirect trauma, in contrast to the direct trauma described above, usually results in the teeth being displaced labially or intruded into the alveolar bone, compared with the unaffected standing teeth.

The displacement again commonly follows one of three movements:

1. A labial movement with fracture of the palatal or lingual alveolar bone and compression of the labial alveolar bone (Fig. 3D).

B

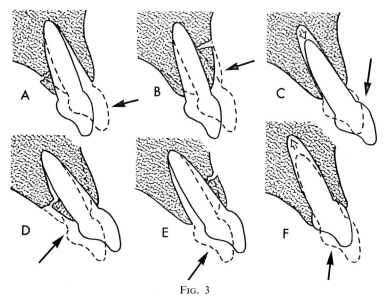

Fig. 3

Types of tooth displacement following direct and indirect trauma.

2. A labial movement with fracture of the labial alveolar bone (Fig. 3E).
3. Intrusion of the tooth into its socket compressing bone in the periapical region, the tooth appearing short on clinical examination (Fig. 3F).

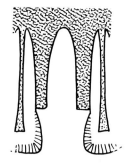

Total Displacement due to Trauma

Total displacement of anterior teeth can also occur. Nearly always the cause of such displacement is the consequence of direct trauma (Fig. 4).

Fig. 4

Total tooth displacement following trauma.

Fracture due to Trauma

Fracture of anterior teeth is a common sequela of a blow to the face. The teeth may be fractured and also show one of the partial displacements listed above. The varieties of fracture fall into four basic types which are the same for both permanent and deciduous dentitions (Fig. 5).

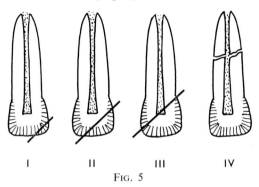

I   II   III   IV

FIG. 5

Classification of tooth fracture.

Type I   Simple fracture of the crown not involving dentine.
Type II Extensive fracture of the crown involving both enamel and dentine but not exposing the dental pulp.
Type III Extensive fracture of the crown exposing the dental pulp.
Type IV Fracture of the root, with or without coronal fracture.

CLASSIFICATION OF TRAUMA TO ANTERIOR TEETH

For treatment purposes the displacement of the tooth can be considered in relation to fracture, if this has occurred, and as an aid to treatment the following simplified classification of trauma to anterior teeth has been devised and will be used throughout this book.

Class I   No fracture or fracture of enamel only, with or without displacement of the tooth.
Class II Fracture of the crown involving both enamel and dentine without exposure of the pulp and with or without displacement of the tooth.
Class III Fracture of the crown exposing the pulp, with or without displacement of the tooth.
Class IV Fracture of the root with or without coronal fracture, with or without displacement of the tooth.
Class V   Total displacement of the tooth.

REFERENCES

BRAUER, J. C. (1964). *Dentistry for Children*, 5th ed. New York. McGraw-Hill.

ELLIS, R. G. (1960). *The Classification and Treatment of Injuries to the Teeth of Children*, 4th ed. Chicago: Year Book Publishers.

HALLETT, G. E. M. (1953). Problems of common interest to the paedodontist and orthodontist with special reference to traumatised incisor cases. *Trans. Eur. orthod. Soc.* 266.

HARDWICK, J. L. & NEWMAN, P. A. (1954). Some observations on the incidence and emergency treatment of fractured permanent anterior teeth of children. *J. dent. Res.* **33**, 730.

HORSNELL, A. M. (1952). Trauma to the incisor teeth. *Br. dent. J.* **93**, 105.

SCHREIBER, C. K. (1959). The effect of trauma on the anterior deciduous teeth. *Br. dent. J.* **106**, 340.

SWEET, C. A. (1942). Fractured anterior permanent teeth. *J. Am. dent. Ass.* **29**, 97.

WORLD HEALTH ORGANIZATION (1957). Accidents in childhood. *Tech. Rep. Ser. Wld Hlth Org.* No. 118.

ZANDER, H. A. & LAW, D. B. (1942). Pulp management in fractures of young permanent teeth. *J. Am. dent. Ass.* **29**, 737.

CHAPTER 2

Assessment of Injury with Aims and Principles of Treatment

THE patient presenting at the surgery following injury to the teeth should have a careful history taken prior to the clinical examination. This should include personal details together with the usual medical and dental history. In recording information about the injury itself, details relating to cause, place and time are particularly relevant.

Cause. The cause of the injury will frequently provide a guide as to whether the injury has been sustained by a direct or an indirect blow.

Place. The place where the accident occurred may provide essential information on the possibility of contamination, such as might occur on the playing-field or in road accidents.

Time. The time of the injury is important in assessing the interval between injury and the commencement of treatment, information which directly affects both the type of treatment to be given and the prognosis.

Pain, if present, should be noted. Absence of pain, however, can be misleading and should not be relied upon in making a diagnosis, since the patient may be in a state of general or local clinical shock. If the patient is in a state of general clinical shock or has suffered a severe injury, he should be treated for this immediately and returned home or to hospital under medical supervision; local treatment of the traumatised teeth should be temporarily delayed.

The recording of data is essential in making a sound treatment plan. A special injury form is advisable, which will ensure the collection of all relevant details in a rapid and logical way. An example of such a form is shown in Figure 6.

The clinical examination should be both extra- and intra-oral. The extra-oral examination should take particular note of any external lacerations to the face and lips (Fig. 7). The intra-oral examination must be a systematic examination of both soft and hard tissues.

TRAUMA CASE HISTORY CHART

1. Name .... Date of Birth..

2. Address.. Age ....

     .... Date of Examination............................. ....

HISTORY OF INJURY

1. Date .... Time ....

2. Time elapsed before examination.. ....

3. Cause and place of injury....... ....

4. Any previous injury to this or other teeth :

5. Patient's symptoms :

CLINICAL EXAMINATION

1. Soft tissue involvement
2. Jaw injuries
    Nose injuries
3. Tooth involvement
     (a) Fracture type

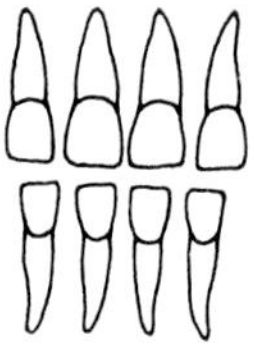

Trauma Classification
Class I
Class II
Class III
Class IV
Class V

     (b) Mobility
     (c) Percussion
     (d) Colour
     (e) Response to vitality testing

cold
heat
electric pulp tester

4. X-ray examination
5. Occlusion   (a) Angle
                 (b) Incisal relationship
6. Treatment already given :

TREATMENT PLAN

Fig. 6
Form suitable for recording relevant trauma details.

A visual and digital examination should be made, followed by other subsidiary aids as are necessary, such as radiographic examinations and tooth vitality tests.

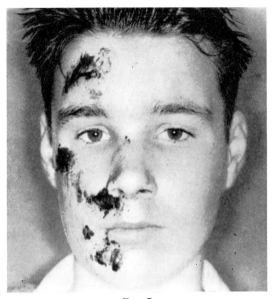

FIG. 7

Associated soft tissue damage in a boy suffering injury to the teeth.

The visual examination should check the following factors:

1. The ability of the child to open his mouth fully, to check damage to the jaws or tempero-mandibular joint.
2. Occlusion both in centric and functional positions, which could be disturbed by tooth displacement.
3. Fractured or missing teeth.
4. Discoloured teeth—transillumination for pulpal congestion is useful.
5. The general dental condition of the patient in respect of caries, gingival inflammation, previous treatment and oral hygiene.
6. Swellings or sinus development, suggesting pulpal death of the traumatised teeth.
7. Bruising or laceration of the soft tissues.

The digital examination should check the following points:

1. Mobility of the teeth.—This is readily estimated by placing a finger behind each tooth in turn and gently pressing the labial surface with a finger of the other hand (Fig. 8). Sometimes it is found that several teeth move together; this may indicate a fracture of the alveolar process.

2. Tenderness on percussion.—This is detected by gently tapping the incisal edges of the teeth with the forefinger. Heavy tapping of the tooth with a dental instrument should be avoided.

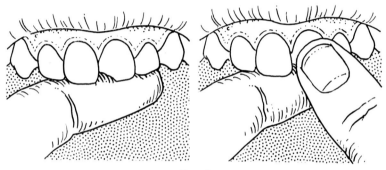

Fig. 8

Method of digital examination to check tooth mobility.

As mentioned above, the two most important subsidiary examinations are radiographic examination and vitality tests.

The radiographic examination is completed by intra-oral periapical radiographs. Alveolar bone and tooth root fractures can be confirmed. The degree of apical development of tooth roots may be ascertained and any pre-existing periapical infection or destruction detected. Displacements and intrusions of the teeth in their sockets can also be checked. Jaw fractures need a full radiographic analysis and such cases should be transferred to an oral surgery unit as soon as possible.

Occasionally a fractured piece of tooth may enter and be retained in the lip. A swollen lip should always be suspect (Allen, 1961) and a radiograph of the lip region should be taken for detection of possible penetration and retention of a piece of fractured tooth (Fig. 9). Chapter 3 deals in more detail with radiographs as an aid to diagnosis.

Vitality tests are helpful, but in the early stages of injury to teeth are of doubtful diagnostic value and may even be mis-leading as the teeth often give a negative response because of local shock. Concussion of the pulp can persist for several weeks with pulpal response gradually returning to normal. Pulp testing at this later time is important when comparison can be made with adjacent uninjured teeth. Thermal testing can be carried out with hot gutta-percha for the effect of heat, with ethyl chloride for cold stimulation (Mumford, 1964*a*), or by electric pulp testing—E.P.T. (Mumford, 1964*b*).

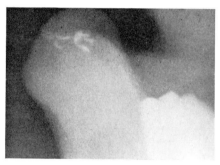

FIG. 9
Radiograph of retained tooth fragments in the
lower lip following tooth fracture.

In making any of these vitality tests, the response of a tooth is checked against the response of an unaffected tooth near to it in the arch. If the response to pulp testing is negative 6 weeks after the injury, the tooth can be considered non-vital. Teeth may die several weeks or even months after injury and checks should be undertaken at six-monthly intervals for 2 years following the trauma.

Classification of the injury can now be made, following the examination, as a guide to treatment required.

PROGNOSIS

Injuries involving the mouth can at first sight appear rather severe, particularly when associated with trauma to the soft tissues. Fortunately, however, most injuries can be adequately treated and fractured or displaced teeth retained and restored to function within a relatively short period. Few traumatised teeth require extraction.

At the first visit, therefore, the management should verge on the conservative side, due considerations being given to the advantages to be gained by retaining teeth even if in occasional cases this is for a few years only.

AIMS AND PRINCIPLES OF TREATMENT

Children who present at the surgery with injuries to the anterior teeth frequently do so as emergencies. The psychological impact of these injuries on the patient and his parent should never be underestimated. Both are upset by the immediate

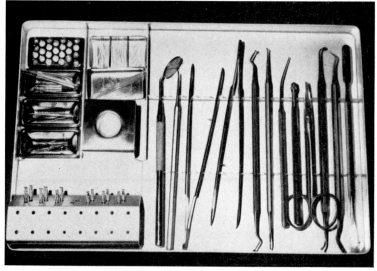

FIG. 10

A suitable instrument tray for emergency treatment of traumatised teeth.

condition and the parent is often anxious about the prognosis, particularly from the point of view of appearance. Unless the practice is adequately prepared to accept such emergencies, lack of professional calm, confidence and competence will serve only to aggravate an already difficult situation.

Since a favourable prognosis is directly related to the interval between the time of injury and the commencement of treatment, injuries should always be seen as soon as possible after the event, even at the expense of deferring treatment for another patient.

It follows that good management of such cases depends

primarily on two factors, firstly, a thorough knowledge of the subject and secondly, a surgery fully prepared to proceed to immediate treatment of both hard and soft tissues. To this end, a sterile receptacle containing a selection of suitable instruments and medicaments should always be maintained in a state of readiness (Fig. 10). Nothing serves to reassure and encourage both patient and parent better than the confidence inspired by a well-prepared dental team.

The aim in any treatment of trauma to the anterior teeth of children should be to maintain the vitality of the injured tooth and to allow normal development of jaws and teeth to proceed. Treatment can, therefore, readily be divided into three catagories: emergency, intermediate restorative and permanent restorative (Table II).

TABLE II

Emergency	Intermediate Restorative	Permanent Restorative
(Immediate Therapy) This aims at keeping the vitality of the fractured or displaced tooth, by protection of the damaged area, treatment of exposed pulp tissue and reduction with immobilisation if the tooth is displaced.	Following a period of rest, if the fractured or displaced tooth remains vital, the fracture can be restored with an aesthetic restoration requiring minimum preparation during the growth and development of the child. This will serve the child until a final restoration can be achieved. If the tooth becomes non-vital, pulp therapy must also be completed.	The placement of a permanent restoration, for example a jacket crown, should not be undertaken before growth has ceased and occlusion established or before gingival contour is stable following active eruption and the pulp safeguarded by adequate dentine formation.

Emergency treatment provides 'first aid' following the injury. The patient must be examined and treated for both general and local injury and infection. As mentioned earlier in the assessment of injury, if the patient is in a general state of clinical shock or has suffered severe injury he should be treated for this immediately and returned to his home or hospital under medical supervision, the local treatment of the traumatised teeth being temporarily delayed.

Consideration must also be given to the place of injury in

respect of tetanus infection; for example, a child suffering trauma on the football field with soft tissue lacerations and tooth fracture should have preventive measures against tetanus given as soon as possible (Convery, 1966). This is best undertaken by the general medical practitioner who will have records of the child's immunisation programme.

Simple soft-tissue lacerations of the mucosa of the lip or tongue can be readily treated by suturing with 000 silk using a $\frac{3}{8}$ or $\frac{1}{2}$ circle 16 mm. atraumatic cutting needle. Severe soft tissue lacerations or jaw fractures should be hospitalised immediately following 'first-aid' treatment.

The majority of tooth fractures or displacements are simple and involve no associated severe injury.

If no tooth fracture or tooth loss has occurred, intermediate restorative or permanent restorative stages may not be necessary. Intermediate restorative dentistry is designed to maintain the vitality of the tooth, to allow normal occlusal and tooth development of the child and to provide an aesthetic restoration. Severe interference caused by the removal of undue tooth tissue in the preparation of a young traumatised tooth could result in pulpal death.

The permanent restoration should only be undertaken when main growth has ceased and occlusion is established. This is not advised before 17 years of age, by which time the gingival contour is usually stable and dentine development is sufficiently advanced to allow a substantial preparation without risk of pulpal exposure.

The treatment will be planned from the information gained at the initial examination. The programme of treatment should always be outlined to the parent at this stage since final success is dependent in no small measure on informed parental co-operation in the months that lie ahead.

REFERENCES

ALLEN, F. J. (1961). Incisor fragments in the lips. *Dent. Practnr. dent. Rec.* **11**, 390.

CONVERY, L. P. (1966). Tetanus prophylaxis for the child with soft tissue injury—the dentist's responsibility. *J. Indianapolis dent. Soc.* **21**, 11.

MUMFORD, J. M. (1964a). Evaluation of gutta-percha and ethyl chloride in pulp testing. *Br. dent. J.* **116**, 338.

MUMFORD, J. M. (1964b). Electric vitality tester. *Dent. Radiogr. Photogr.* **37**, 75.

CHAPTER 3

Radiographs as an Aid to Diagnosis

RADIOGRAPHIC evidence in the management of traumatised anterior teeth is of value in determining the presence of alveolar or root fracture, the size of the pulpal tissue and its relationship to the line of fracture, the condition of the periapical tissues, and the developmental stage of the root. It also forms a valuable record for later comparison.

Recognition of the abnormal depends largely on the knowledge of the normal anatomical structures and their variation due to radiographic technique.

Consider first the upper jaw in the inter-canine region. The median suture of the palate is readily identified between the two central incisors as a thin, dark (radiolucent) line bounded by two thin white (radio-opaque) lines (Fig. 11). These radio-opaque lines may not be so clearly defined if 'struck' by divergent rays as when the centre ray is positioned nearer a lateral incisor (compare Fig. 12A and B).

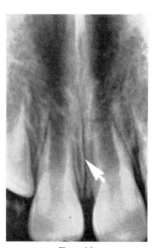

FIG. 11
Median suture.

The incisive canal (anterior palatine canal) is situated between the roots of the two upper central incisor teeth and appears as an area of increased radiolucency in the cancellous bone (Fig. 13). Because of its position close to the apices, radiographic technique may project it over the periapical region, giving rise to misinterpretation (Figs 14 and 15).

The upper part of the incisive canal unites with two small canals, the naso-palatine, one on each side, which emerge on the nasal cavity floor close to the nasal septum (Fig. 16). Radiographs taken with the X-ray tube centred over the lateral

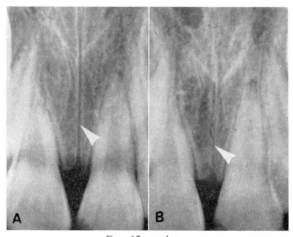

Fig. 12a and b
The effect of change in tube position in respect of the median
suture.

incisor and canine region frequently show the entrance to the
naso-palatine canal as a very dark, well-defined radiolucent
area in the floor of the nose (Figs 17 and 18). From the orifice,
a faint radiolucency, often bounded by faint lines of cortical
bone, curves towards the mesial aspect of the central incisor

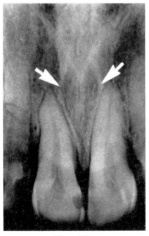

Fig. 13
Incisive canal.

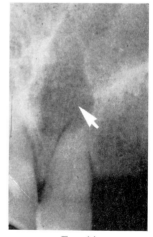

Fig. 14
Incisive canal foramen.

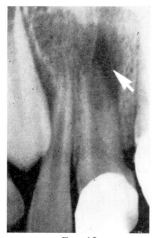

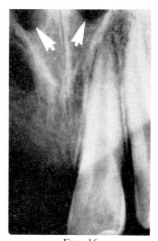

FIG. 15
Periapical rarefaction, maxillary right central incisor.

FIG. 16
Naso-palatine foramina.

apex, but occasionally is projected over it and may lead to confusion in interpretation (Fig. 19).

The floor of the nasal cavities curves forward to end in the midline as a sharp projection, the anterior nasal spine, situated above and between the central incisors. On radiographs, the

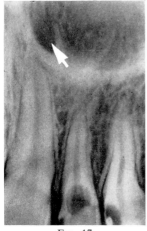

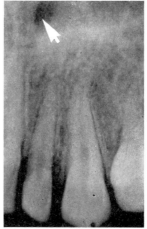

FIG. 17
Naso-palatine foramen.

FIG. 18
Naso-palatine foramen.

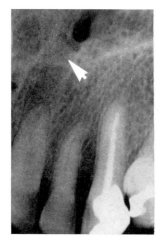

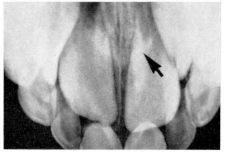

FIG. 20
Anterior nasal spine.

FIG. 19
Naso-palatine foramen and canal.

anterior limit of the nasal floor and spine shows as two thin, curved radio-opaque lines which unite over the median suture. On intra-oral radiographs, the relationship between the anterior nasal spine and the apices of the central incisors may vary (Figs 20 to 22). In some cases it may appear well clear of the apices and its recognition is relatively simple. On the other hand, it may be projected between the apices or further down between

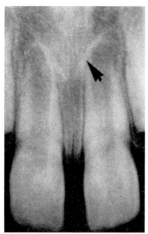

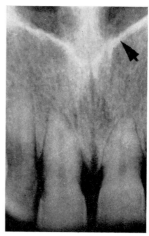

FIG. 21
Anterior nasal spine.

FIG. 22
Anterior nasal spine.

the roots, bringing the radiolucency of the nasal floor over or near the apices, and thus suggesting the presence of a diffuse periapical rarefaction. Figure 23A gives the appearance of an extensive diffuse periapical rarefaction in relation to the upper right central incisor. The anterior nasal spine is projected over the apices of the upper central incisors and the radiolucency may be due to the floor of the nasal cavity. The radiograph shown in Figure 23B supports this suggestion as the changed viewpoint no longer shows the extensive radiolucent area.

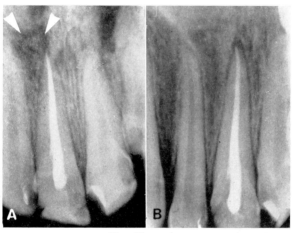

FIG. 23A and B

A suggests periapical rarefaction, maxillary right central incisor; B, altered tube position suggests radiolucent area was due to floor of nasal cavity.

Cancellous bone on a radiograph appears as small, irregular, dark (radiolucent) areas (the marrow spaces) bounded by thin plates of bone. The size of these spaces may be altered by technique. They will appear slightly increased in size if the distance between the bone and the film is increased while the tube position remains unchanged. Increasing the distance of the tube will reduce them to nearer their correct size (Fig. 24 A and B).

Apparent changes in anatomical structure such as those described above may occur if the radiographic technique is altered from that of holding the film close to the palate with the finger, to one where the periapical film is held horizontally

C

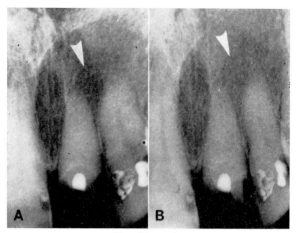

Fig. 24A and B

Effect of technique on the size of the marrow spaces in cancellous bone.

between the upper and lower incisors. In the finger method of holding the film, with the vertical angle of the tube at 45° and the centre ray directed to strike the root about 4 mm. apical to the cervical margin, the cone is close to the tip of the nose.

In the periapical occlusal view, however, with the vertical angle at 55° the tube position will require to be altered relative to the nose so that the centre ray strikes the root at the same point (Fig. 25). This technique provides a very useful alter-

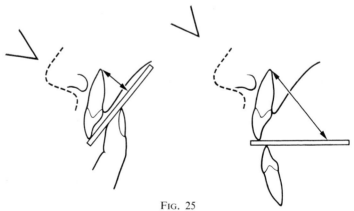

Fig. 25

Relative position of the tube cone to nose, with film held to palate and film in occlusal position.

native periapical view provided it is remembered to alter the tube position to compensate for the changed relationship between the apices and film.

In anterior radiographs of the maxilla, faint opacities, usually with well-defined margins, due to shadows thrown by the cartilage of the nose, are occasionally seen. The outlines of the nares, or nostrils, also produce margins on intra-oral films which may not always be readily recognised as originating from the nasal structures.

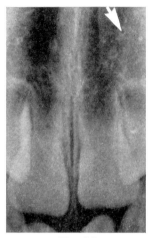

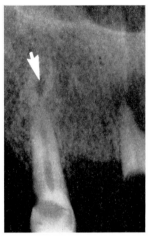

<table>
<tr><td>Fig. 26
Foramina of nutrient canals.</td><td>Fig. 27
Nutrient canal superimposed over the apex of maxillary right canine.</td></tr>
</table>

The cancellous bone is traversed by numerous small vessels which, in the dry skull, show as small foramina in the cortical layer, generally on the crests of the inter-dental bone and in the palate. These small channels are referred to as nutrient canals. Figure 26 illustrates an example of foramina occurring in the palatal area. In the anterior region of the maxilla these canals are not usually of sufficient size to produce prominent radiolucent areas. However, they may sometimes be more readily seen in the lateral, canine and premolar regions, where, as radiolucent lines, they may be confused with fractured alveolar bone, fractured roots or periapical lesions. Figure 27 shows a canal superimposed over the periapical region of the upper right canine. Notice the radio-opacity of the peripheral cortical layer of bone forming the canal. Sometimes the foramen can be recognised by careful study of the cortical layer at the periphery where the canals may be seen leading to them. Figure 28A and B are two views of the same case. Figure 28A shows a large prominent foramen in the apical region of the upper left canine, while Figure 28B shows the radiolucent canal leading to the foramen, thus avoiding the possibility of a misdiagnosis.

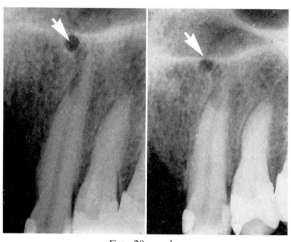

FIG. 28A and B

A shows a large prominent foramen in the apical region, maxillary left canine; B shows radiolucent canal leading to foramen, eliminating possibility of mis-diagnosis.

Nutrient canals are more often to be found in the mandibular incisor region. Here, they form well-defined radiolucent lines which run vertically in the inter-dental bone towards the inter-dental crests (Fig. 29).

Other small canals that may be seen are those running to the apices of teeth. Again, these are more likely to be seen in relation to the mandibular incisors. Their presence shows on a radiograph as prominent, thin, radio-opaque lines of cortical bone leading to the apices of the teeth (Fig. 30).

The bone surrounding the roots at the cervical margin may sometimes be represented on the radiograph as two margins, one the level of the alveolar bone on the palatal or lingual aspect, and the other, the level of alveolar bone on the labial side.

Some radiographs may show the bone level crossing the roots as a single margin.

Surrounding the roots and continuing over the crest of the inter-dental bone is the lamina dura, a narrow opaque line due to a thin layer of cortical bone (Fig. 31). This shows more readily in some areas than others. The lower anterior teeth have oval or flat-sided roots and hence these teeth will more easily show the lamina dura. Upper central incisors, on the

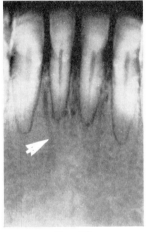

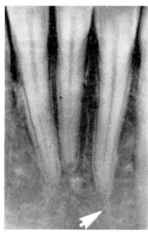

Fig. 29
Nutrient canals in the mandibular incisor region.

Fig. 30
Canals leading to apices of teeth.

other hand, with their conoid roots, do not always show the presence of the lamina dura. Figure 32 shows the presence of the lamina dura, Figure 33 does not.

Between the lamina dura and the root is the dark, radiolucent line formed by the periodontal membrane (Fig. 34). Knowledge of the normal appearance of both the lamina dura and the periodontal space is of importance in diagnosing a deviation from the normal.

In the upper jaw, where the opacity of the anterior margin of the nasal floor may sometimes be thrown over the apices of the central incisors, so in the mandible the opacity of the mental ridge may occur over the apices of the mandibular incisors. This opacity is more noticeable and prominent in cases where the mental ridge is well developed. It appears on a radiograph

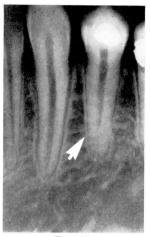

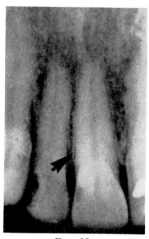

FIG. 31
Lamina dura associated with mandibular teeth.

FIG. 32
Lamina dura associated with maxillary teeth.

as two broad radio-opaque lines, superimposed over or near the apices of the incisors, meeting in the midline (Fig. 35).

Misleading artefacts may sometimes be introduced in radiographs. These occur either by excessive pressure from the incisal edges of the teeth while holding the film in the occlusal position or by pressure from the finger-nail while opening the film packet in the dark room. In the first case, a radiolucent

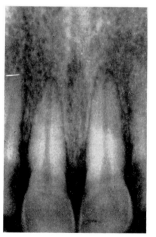

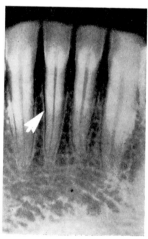

FIG. 33
Apparent absence of lamina dura associated with maxillary teeth.

FIG. 34
Periodontal membrane.

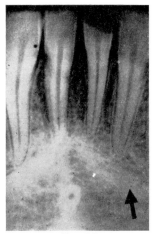

FIG. 35
Mental ridge.

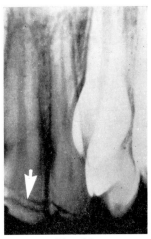

FIG. 36
Apparent fracture lines in maxillary left central and lateral incisors due to biting on film.

line appears over the crown and gives a very realistic appearance of fracture (Fig. 36). Viewing the film horizontally will show a kink in the surface. The second case generally appears as a slightly curved, small radiolucent line over a root (Figs 37 and 38). Frequently, this shows as an obvious artefact, but may not always be immediately evident. Again, viewing the film in the horizontal position will reveal the origin.

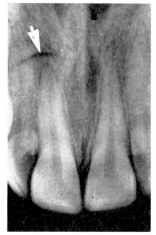

FIG. 37
Artefact due to finger nail pressure on film.

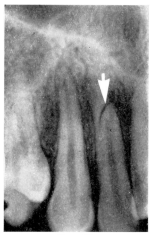

FIG. 38
Artefact due to finger nail pressure on film.

Diagnosis of Root Fracture

In cases of suspected root fracture, the normal radiographic periapical techniques are generally used. It should be borne in mind, however, that the fracture appearance may be modified by two factors:

1. The direction of the X-rays to the fracture;
2. The direction or plane of the fracture itself.

A few simple experiments will demonstrate the changes in radiographic appearance brought about by the divergence of the beam and the position of the centre ray to the object.

A post-card for example, may be radio-opaque or radiolucent, depending on the manner in which it is radiographed (Fig. 39). If the post-card is arranged at 90° to the film and the centre ray positioned to pass through the edge of the card (Fig. 41), then

Figs 39–50

Experimental evidence of radiographic differences caused by altering the position of the dental cone.

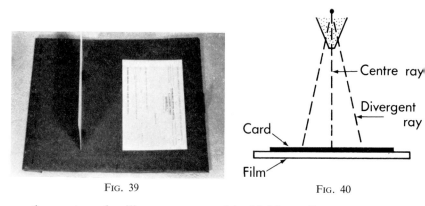

FIG. 39   FIG. 40

the post-card will appear as a thin highly radio-opaque line (Fig. 42). If the experiment is repeated, with the tube moved so that the centre ray narrowly misses the edge of the card (Fig. 43) two changes occur; firstly, the radio-opacity is much reduced, and secondly, the previously thin opaque line becomes much wider (Fig. 44). This is due to the divergent rays striking the flat surface of the card and the centre ray missing it entirely. On the other hand (Fig. 40) the same post-card placed parallel to the film appears completely radiolucent. Hence the card will be radio-opaque or radiolucent depending on the direction of the X-ray beam relative to it.

FIGS 39–50 (*continued*)

Experimental evidence of radiographic differences caused by altering the position of the dental cone.

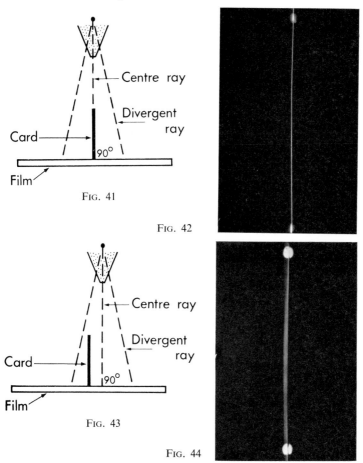

FIG. 41

FIG. 42

FIG. 43

FIG. 44

A dental example of this may occur with flat-sided or oval roots, such as the lower incisors, which, if rotated through 90°, may not appear on the radiograph. Their place on the film is apparently taken by the overlying cancellous bone structure (Figs 45 to 47).

A tooth fracture generally appears at maximum radiolucency when the centre ray passes directly through it. This can be

FIGS 39–50 (*continued*)

Experimental evidence of radiographic differences caused by altering the position of the dental cone.

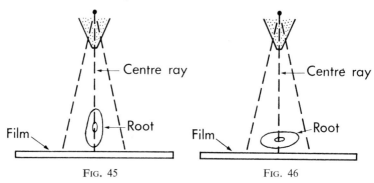

FIG. 45   FIG. 46

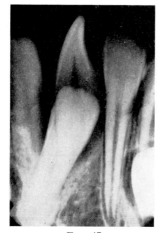

FIG. 47

illustrated by using a piece of ply-wood divided into two pieces by a diagonal cut and then joined in position again by Sellotape. The wood is then radiographed with the centre ray in two positions (Fig. 48):

1. At 90° to the wood surface;
2. With the centre ray passing directly along the diagonal cut.

The first radiograph (Fig. 49) does not reveal the break in continuity in the wood, since the degree of opacity at points 'A' and 'D' in Figure 48 is identical. On the other hand, if the centre ray is repositioned to follow the diagonal cut the resulting radiograph shows a definite break in continuity (Fig. 50).

By cutting roots of teeth in various planes and radiographing the reassembled pieces, differences in the appearance of the fracture lines can be studied. The radiographic appearance can then be directly related both to the shape of the object, for

FIGS 39–50 (*continued*)

Experimental evidence of radiographic differences caused by altering the position of the dental cone.

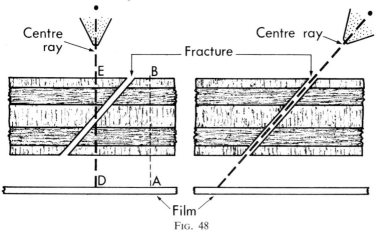

FIG. 48

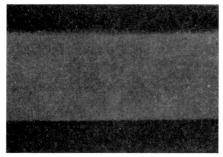

FIG. 49

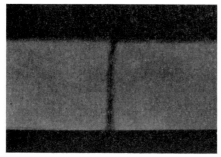

FIG. 50

example, the conoid root of an upper central incisor, and also
to the plane of the cut, by studying the teeth visually.

Figure 51 illustrates the direction of cuts made in maxillary
incisors.

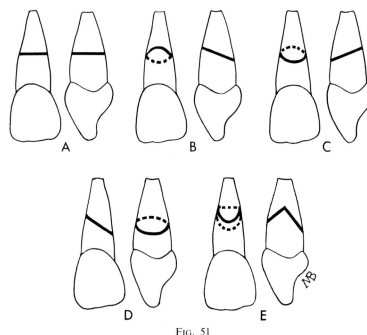

FIG. 51

The direction of experimental cuts in maxillary incisors.

(A) a simple transverse cut at 90° to the long axis of the
tooth;

(B) an oblique labio-palatal cut in a coronal direction;

(C) an oblique labio-palatal cut in an apical direction;

(D) an oblique mesio-distal cut;

(E) an inverted 'V' shaped cut in a labio-palatal direction.

Figures 52 and 53 illustrate the results when these teeth are
reassembled.

In Figure 52A the centre ray has been in line with the fracture
and therefore shows a clearly defined radiolucent line. If,
however, the centre ray does not pass directly through the fracture, then changes in the radiographic appearances occur and
the fracture line will be less well-defined (Fig. 52B).

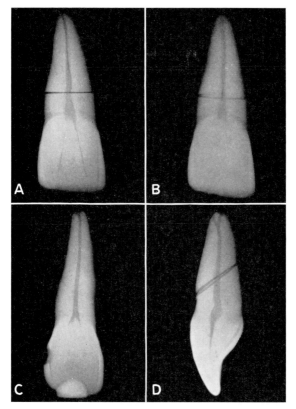

FIG. 52A–D

The radiographic appearances obtained when the sectioned teeth, shown diagrammatically in Figure 51, are reassembled.

If the teeth are fractured obliquely in a labio-palatal direction as illustrated by Figure 51B and C, then a radiograph taken from the labial aspect may fail to define the line of fracture which is only seen as two faint radiolucent lines, curved because of the conoid nature of the root (Fig. 52C). In radiographs taken in the mouth, the fracture lines will be still further obscured by the superimposed trabeculae pattern of the bone. Figure 52D, however, shows the same tooth radiographed from the proximal aspect clearly indicating the labio-palatal fracture line.

When the plane of fracture runs obliquely in a mesio-distal direction the fracture line may be clearly defined (Fig. 53A), or

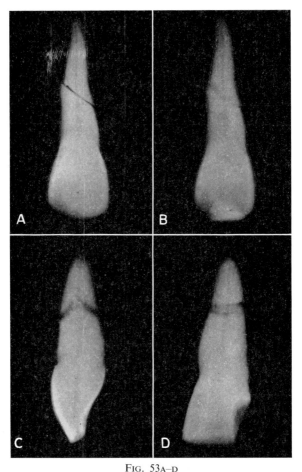

FIG. 53A–D

The radiographic appearances obtained when the sectioned teeth, shown diagrammatically in Fig. 51, are reassembled.

only partially obscured if the centre ray is not directly in line (Fig. 53B). A fracture of this type is, therefore, more likely to be recognised on a radiograph taken in the mouth than the example in Figure 52C.

Figure 53c is a radiograph in a mesio-distal direction to show a fracture taking the form of an inverted 'V'. This introduces three levels, which on a radiograph from the labial aspect (Fig. 53D), show as a wide radiolucent zone with one or more radio-opaque areas crossing it. These radio-opacities give the suggestion that detached fragments of root lie within the fracture line.

If the plane of fracture is not uniform, but has a slight twist, then radiographic appearance shows two radiolucent lines which cross each other in the fashion of a figure '8', again giving the suggestion that a fragment is detached. This is best illustrated in the example of the fractured mandible where the apparently isolated fragment is readily seen (Fig. 54). However, the photograph of the mandible (Fig. 55) clearly shows the nature of the fracture through the outer and inner plates at the angle of the mandible.

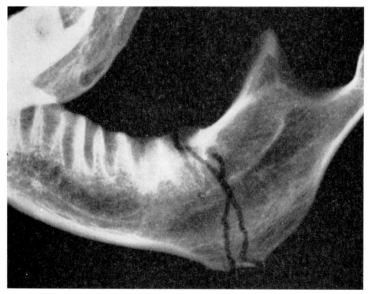

FIG. 54

The radiographic appearance of a figure of '8' fracture of the mandible.

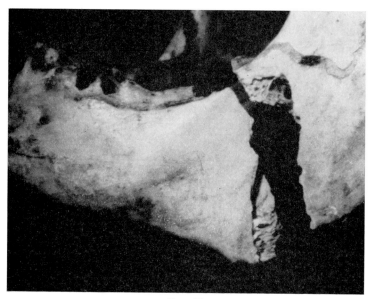

FIG. 55

Photograph of fractured mandible illustrated in Figure 54, showing nature of the fracture.

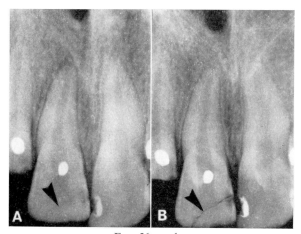

FIG. 56A and B

Fracture of the crown of a maxillary right central incisor. In A the tube is angled at 45° and the film is held to the palate, and in B the tube is angled at 55° and the film is held in occlusal position.

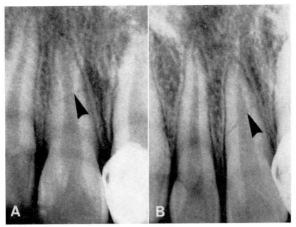

FIG. 57A and B

Root fracture of a maxillary right central incisor. In A the tube
is centred through the right central incisor, and in B the tube is
centred through the right lateral incisor.

From a clinical diagnostic point of view of tooth fracture it is
therefore better that the centre ray passes as nearly as possible
through the fracture line (Fig. 56A and B). In cases of doubt
a radiograph with the centre ray directed through the teeth
adjacent to the suspected tooth should be taken. In this way a
divergent ray entering from the mesial or distal side may show
the presence of a fracture which might otherwise be missed
(Fig. 57A and B).

D

CHAPTER 4

Emergency Treatment

THE aim of emergency treatment is to provide immediate first aid for any or all of the injuries associated with an accident to the face or mouth. These include soft tissue damage, partial displacements, complete tooth loss, crown fractures with or without pulpal exposure and root fractures.

The emergency treatment appropriate to these conditions which may be found in a child who has suffered such an accident and presents at the dental surgery, is discussed in this chapter in order of clinical procedure, depending on the extent of the injury.

EMERGENCY SOFT TISSUE CARE

As outlined in aims and principles of treatment, soft tissue lacerations must be adequately treated. Patients with severe lacerations of the face or oral mucosa should be hospitalised immediately following first-aid care. Minor soft tissue lacerations of the mucosa of the lip or tongue can be readily treated by suturing with 000 silk using a $\frac{3}{8}$ or $\frac{1}{2}$ circle 16 mm. atraumatic cutting needle. These needles and sutures can be purchased in sterile packs and should be available for immediate use, if required, in any dental surgery. Tetanus prophylaxis for a child suffering severe soft tissue injury or puncture wounds in conjunction with tooth damage is the dentist's responsibility. Generally a child is adequately protected from tetanus by active immunisation with a series of injections (normally three) of tetanus toxoid. This toxoid is a formalised preparation of exotoxin, altered so that it causes no illness but produces an adequate level of antibodies. The dentist should arrange for the child to see his family doctor immediately for this protection. If active immunisation has not been undertaken, passive immunisation with tetanus anti-toxin can be commenced. Passive immunisation is itself not without dangers since it may produce anaphylactic shock. Such immunisation should be undertaken only where the past immunisation programme of the child is known. With any of the soft tissue wounds, adequate debridement of the area should be completed as a first-aid measure. Gentle cleansing and irrigation with normal saline will help to reduce the amount of dead tissue and the risk of anaerobic conditions. Surface antiseptics may also be used to reduce the bacterial count, especially of pathogenic staphylococci and streptococci, on the skin or mucosa of the wound site. A suitable antiseptic which can be used is Cetrimide or Cetavlon, a quaternary ammonium compound. A 1 per cent w/v Cetrimide solution BPC, BNF, can be used for wound cleansing. Hibitane (chlorhexidine digluconate) in a 0·5 per cent w/v solution is another useful surface antiseptic which is effective against Gram-positive and Gram-negative organisms.

The parent and child must be instructed to keep the mouth as clean as possible. Saline or sodium bicarbonate mouth washes should be prescribed after meals, for 5 days following the injury.

TREATMENT OF TOOTH DISPLACEMENTS WITH NO ROOT FRACTURE

Before a decision on reimplantation or repositioning of a tooth is taken, a careful assessment of the occlusion should be made, since the space created by the loss of an incisor tooth may be used for general realignment of the anterior segment. This could avoid extractions in the buccal segments at a later date and considerably reduce the period of orthodontic treatment.

If assessment of the mouth as a whole indicates that retaining the displaced tooth would be of advantage to the child, immediate emergency care should be commenced.

Complete Displacement

If the child is seen within 4 to 8 hours of the injury the displaced tooth can be correctly repositioned and immobilised. Experimental work on animals has indicated that the longer that the tooth was out of the mouth the worse would be the result (Flanagan and Myers, 1958; Löe and Waerhaug, 1961). The cause of failure is not inadequate reattachment of the tooth, which is invariably successful, but of progressive root resorption. However, even when root resorption does occur, if the tooth can be maintained in position for several years it acts as an ideal space maintainer during the mixed and early permanent dentition period. At this later date a bridge or denture can be considered if the root resorption is so severe that extraction of the tooth is indicated. Of several techniques described the rationale recently outlined by Bennett (1968) fulfils suitable and essential requirements.

The tooth and socket should be gently cleaned with sterile cotton-wool and gauze soaked in normal saline solution, taking care to retain any adherent periodontal membrane.

If the root is fully formed, the pulp should be removed via the palatal cingulum and a root filling of gutta-percha or silver and a root filling paste inserted. The root should be shortened by 2 to 3 mm. with a stone or disc, smoothing any sharp edges and a retrograde root filling of silver amalgam placed. This apicectomy facilitates repositioning of the tooth without apical pressure, eliminates the apical delta and the retrograde amalgam filling ensures an adequate apical seal. During treatment, if the root is held apex downwards in gauze moistened with saline, the periodontal membrane is neither allowed to dry out nor become contaminated with root filling materials.

If the tooth is immature, no immediate pulp treatment is indicated, but it is essential to keep the tooth under strict observation. Henning (1965) has reimplanted teeth with maintenance of vitality and gives evidence of one case where the root development was incomplete at the time of accident but development continued until apical closure occurred.

Whatever the stage of root development the tooth should be replaced in its socket using gentle finger pressure, taking care to return it to its original position and axial inclination. Local anaesthesia is rarely required to undertake this procedure.

Partial Displacement

If the tooth has been partially displaced, immediate pulp therapy is not indicated unless tooth fracture involving the dental pulp has also occurred. However, in the mature tooth, pulp death will normally occur and root canal therapy should be

commenced as soon as possible after reduction and immobilisation has been achieved.

As with complete tooth displacement mentioned above, the
tooth can be gently repositioned with finger pressure. Anaesthesia is, as before, rarely required to undertake this procedure,
but if the displacement is severe, local or general anaesthesia
can be used to reposition the tooth or teeth in their correct
positions.

Stabilisation of Displaced Teeth

When a tooth has been repositioned, the surface of the crown
should be smeared liberally with petroleum jelly and an alginate
impression taken. The petroleum jelly on the tooth surface
allows easy removal of the impression without moving the
involved tooth. If more than one tooth is loosened, a layer of
thin red casting-wax can be used to cover the surfaces of the
teeth prior to the impression, again to ensure that no pressures
are exerted against the injured teeth during the placing and
removal of the impression material.

From such an impression several types of splint can be made,
all of which are adequate to immobilise the teeth, but in the
cases of close bite or where teeth are missing from the arch,
cast-metal cap splints are advisable. Two teeth either side of a
displaced tooth are necessary for support and if more than two
teeth are loosened a full-arch cap splint is necessary.

In all types of splint described below it is advisable to leave
an area of the palatal surface uncovered for vitality testing,
otherwise it may be necessary to remove the splint prematurely.

As an interim measure, the injured teeth must have a temporary splint constructed until the permanent splint is made.
Such a splint can be fabricated easily from the foil of an
X-ray film packet or from a metal milk-bottle top (Slack and
Birch, 1958). The foil is gently adapted over the tooth surfaces,
trimmed to follow the gingival contour and cemented in place
using a quick-setting zinc oxide and eugenol cement (Fig. 58).
If the pulp of the injured tooth is exposed, this must be treated
prior to cementing the splint. The emergency splint will
usually last two to three days with the zinc oxide and eugenol
cement acting as the immobilising agent. The foil merely
protects the cement from being removed during mastication.

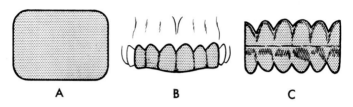

Fɪɢ. 58

Adaptation of radiographic foil to fabricate temporary splint.

A second useful method of temporary stabilisation is coronal wiring. Using soft, stainless steel, or brass ligature wire 0·3 to 0·4 mm. in diameter, the crowns are wired together by either of the two methods illustrated in Figures 59 and 60, taking care not to traumatise the gingivae and ensuring that the free end and interdental ligatures are carefully turned into embrasures to avoid injury to the lips (Fig. 61). This is a particularly useful method of stabilisation prior to impression taking for a permanent splint.

The permanent splint when fitted should be kept in place for 8 to 12 weeks with a preliminary check for vitality some 3 to 4

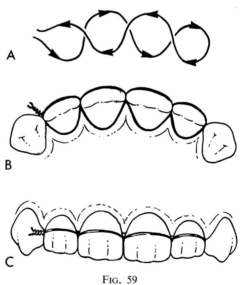

Fɪɢ. 59

Figure of '8' wiring to stabilise loosened teeth.

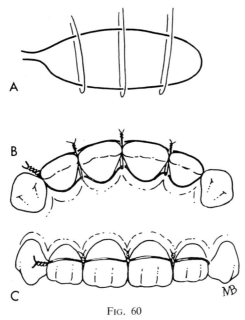

FIG. 60

Essig wiring technique to stabilise loosened teeth.

weeks after injury. If pulpal death of a tooth has occurred, or if a fractured tooth needs additional treatment, pulp therapy and intermediate restorative treatment can be commenced at this time. Even if no other treatment is considered necessary on

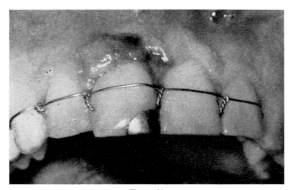

FIG. 61

Clinical photograph of Essig wiring.

removal of the splint, the traumatised teeth should be kept under routine clinical and radiographic check for vitality at six-monthly intervals for a further 2 years since pulpal death may occur during the period following initial displacement.

Of the permanent splints, those made from acrylic resin are probably the most acceptable. Because of their good aesthetic qualities, they help to minimise the psychological trauma to both parent and child and they possess the further advantage of relative ease of construction and minimal loss of clinical time (Fig. 62). Horsnell and Brown (1956) describe a rapid method of constructing such a splint (see Appendix A).

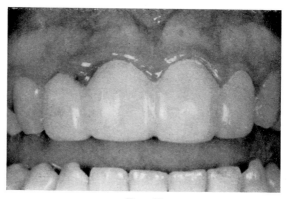

FIG. 62
Acrylic splint illustrating
acceptable appearance.

In cases of maxillary incisor protrusion, as in Angle Class II division I, it is usually only necessary to cap four to six teeth, but in cases of close bite, the splint should cover all the occlusal surfaces. Acrylic splints are cemented in place with quick-setting zinc oxide cements.

Cast silver splints, although less aesthetically pleasing, do provide greater rigidity and can be individually designed to suit the particular requirements of the case. All cast splints should leave the palatal or lingual surfaces uncovered for reasons already given (Fig. 63).

The cast splint is prepared from an alginate or rubber base impression. When cast, the splint should be accurately finished

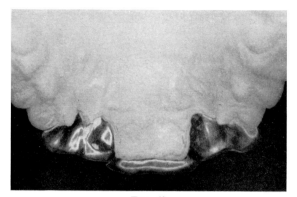

FIG. 63
Palatal view of cast silver splint.

and highly polished to aid oral hygiene (Fig. 64). The method of construction is described in Appendix B. The splint is cemented in place with Ames black copper cement and left in place for 8 to 12 weeks.

In severe injuries, particularly those involving teeth with closed apices, pulpal death is a common sequel. This may occur rapidly or more slowly over a prolonged period of time, and therefore regular vitality testing and periodic radiographic examination must be maintained.

The Orthodontic Splint. This splint suffers from a number of

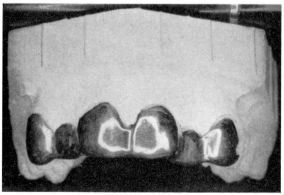

FIG. 64
Completed silver splint in position on model.

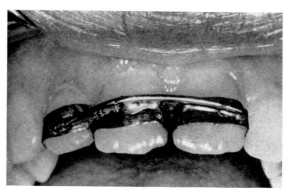

FIG. 65
Orthodontic splint.

disadvantages which limit its usefulness. A high degree of patient co-operation is required in a somewhat lengthy procedure which may result in additional damage to the involved tissues. The orthodontic splint is not suited to young patients, since it is particularly susceptible to damage, and good oral hygiene is not always maintained. Nevertheless, it has a place in stabilisation procedures and is particularly useful in reimplantation, where the totally displaced tooth can be banded outside the mouth (Fig. 65).

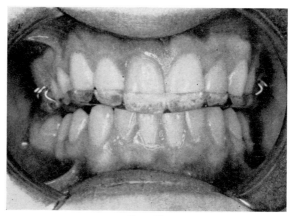

FIG. 66
Removable splint of Sved type.

Removable Splints. Removable splints are of value in stabilising mobile teeth where only minor displacement has occurred. They have the disadvantage that they are under the control of the child, and may therefore be removed at will, although from the oral hygiene point of view this may prove to be an advantage (Fig. 66).

Some Methods of Bite Relief. In occlusions where a close bite exists, it is frequently necessary to protect the injured tooth,

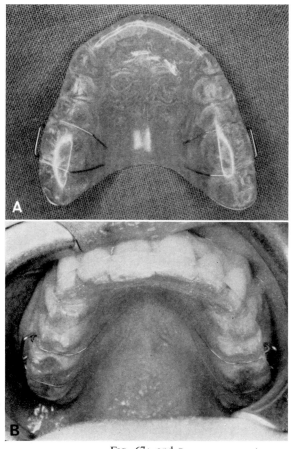

FIG. 67A and B

Bite relief by capping the cheek teeth. A shows completed splint, B shows splint in position in the mouth.

or teeth, from further stress by relieving the bite. In some cases this may be achieved by minimal incisal grinding of the injured or opposing incisors with a disc or stone. More commonly, the bite is relieved by the placement of a removable appliance which caps the cheek teeth in either the mandibular or maxillary arches (Fig. 67).

Immediate Treatment Class I Injuries

Although Class I injuries may involve only minimal loss of enamel or indeed no loss whatever, such injuries should never be regarded as trivial, since degenerative changes in the pulp may subsequently occur. Such changes are more likely in mature teeth with closed apices, because of the greater danger to the pulpal blood vessels. In the immature tooth with a wide-open apex pulpal death is unlikely to result from damage to the pulpal blood vessels except in cases of gross displacement. Ellis (1960) believes that traumatised teeth which do not fracture suffer greater pulpal damage than teeth which do, because the energy expended in fracture is not transmitted to the pulp or surrounding structures.

It is essential, therefore, that a thorough clinical examination is carried out as previously outlined, embracing both adjacent and opposing teeth and including intra-oral radiographs.

Radiographs are essential for the following reasons:

1. To establish the developmental stage of the root;
2. To determine the size of the pulp and its relationship to the line of fracture;
3. To eliminate the possibility of root fracture;
4. To assess possible damage to the supporting structures;
5. For record purposes and later comparison.

In the absence of soft tissue injuries or displacements the immediate treatment is limited to the smoothing of any sharp enamel edges, taking care to avoid the generation of heat which might add to the pulpal irritation. A period of watchful waiting follows during which the patient will be recalled at regular intervals for vitality checks and radiographic examinations. Initially these re-examinations should take place at monthly intervals for the first 3 months, then at three-monthly intervals for a further 6 months and thereafter at the routine six-monthly visit.

The parents should be advised about possible sequelae before dismissing the patient at the initial visit.

Immediate Treatment Class II Injuries

Class II fractures with loss of enamel and dentine require immediate attention to avoid further damage to the pulp from thermal shock and bacterial infiltration of the exposed dentinal tubules. Fortunately, many patients with Class II injuries, unlike those with Class I injuries, report to the dentist early, usually because of pain from thermal changes.

A full clinical and radiographic examination is the immediate requirement. Once the classification has been established soft tissue injuries and displacements are dealt with first.

Three factors govern the treatment of Class II fractures:
1. The time dentine has been left exposed;
2. The remaining thickness of the dentine between fracture surface and pulp;
3. The stage of development of the root.

Recent Injuries. In Class II cases, provided injury is recent and does not involve a near exposure, the immediate treatment is to cover the exposed dentinal tubules by applying a dressing of calcium hydroxide paste to the exposed dentine. This is followed by a thin mix of oxyphosphate cement which is allowed to set before fitting a suitable retainer for the dressing.

A successful retainer must satisfy two essential requirements. Firstly, it must restore the anatomical form of the crown so that contact points, if lost, are re-established and so that the tooth remains under the same soft tissue influence as before the fracture. Secondly, it must remain in place for the required length of time, a minimum period of 8 to 12 weeks.

While a cellulose acetate crown form is perhaps the simplest to adapt, is aesthetically pleasing and meets the first requirement, it is not generally well retained and is susceptible to wear. The essential of emergency treatment is to ensure that the pulp of the traumatised tooth is afforded every opportunity for recovery, and aesthetics should not be an all-important factor since this phase of the treatment is of relatively short duration.

A suitable retainer can readily be fashioned from a copper impression ring. The mesio-distal width of the tooth is measured with a pair of dividers and a ring of suitable size selected.

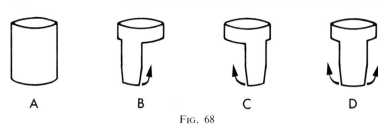

A   B   C   D

FIG. 68

Method of adapting copper ring as a temporary retainer for immediate protection: A untrimmed ring; B ring trimmed for mesio-incisal angle fracture;
C ring trimmed for disto-incisal angle fracture; D ring trimmed for horizontal
fracture of incisal edge.

The ring, which need not be annealed, is then cut to the required
pattern (Fig. 68) and the edges smoothed with a finishing stone.
Using a pair of Johnson or other contouring pliers, the retainer
is then gently adapted to the tooth and the incisal flap turned
under and tucked beneath the lingual portion.   The cap so
formed is cemented in place with oxyphosphate cement (Fig. 69).

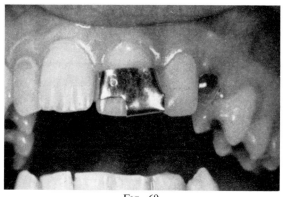

FIG. 69

Clinical photograph of copper ring retainer in position,
protecting a disto-incisal angle fracture.

A second and equally satisfactory method, but requiring a
spot welder, is the fabrication of a cap from orthodontic stainless
steel tape 3 mm. wide by 0·8 mm. thick (Figs 70 and 71).

Pre-formed stainless steel crowns (Fig. 72), however, are now
considered the method of choice (Barrie and Hargreaves, 1969).
The tooth to be fitted is measured with a pair of dividers and a

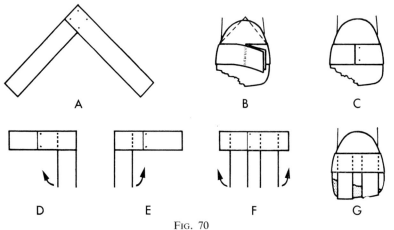

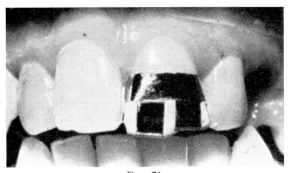

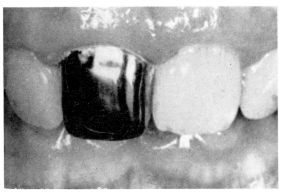

Fig. 70

Fabrication of temporary retainer from stainless steel tape. D, E and F illustrate the position of vertical tapes in relation to position of fractured tooth surface.

Fig. 71

Clinical photograph of stainless steel retainer in position.

Fig. 72

Pre-formed stainless steel crown in position in the mouth.

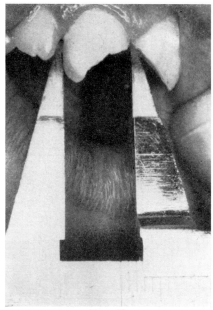

FIG. 73
Tooth measurement for crown selection.

crown of suitable size selected (Fig. 73).   With a pair of curved
crown shears it is cut to the required length and correct gingival
contour.   The cut edges are smoothed and the periphery contoured with contouring pliers to provide a spring fit.   In order
to aid adaptation and avoid pressure when fitting, the palatal
surface is perforated with a No. 3 round bur (Fig. 74).   If

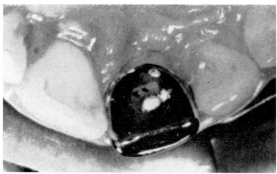

FIG. 74
Palatal perforation of stainless steel crown.

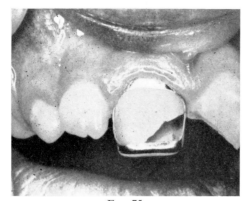

FIG. 75
Labial face of stainless steel crown cut away prior
to facing.

thought desirable, the appearance of this crown can be improved
by cutting out the labial surface and, after placement, adding a
silicate or acrylic facing of suitable shade (Figs 75 and 76).

Whatever type of retainer is fitted it is necessary to check the

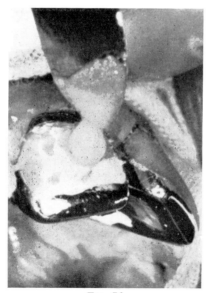

FIG. 76
Application of acrylic facing to stainless
steel crown.

occlusion. This is done with the retainer in place before cementation. In close bite conditions it may be necessary to relieve biting pressure upon the fractured tooth. When the fracture is complicated by displacement the fitted splint can serve as an excellent retainer for any dressing.

In Class II injuries, where the thickness of dentine between the fractured surface and the pulp is thin, the case should be regarded as one of pulpal exposure and treated as a Class III injury. Attempts to pulp cap such injuries even if the injury is recent and the apex wide open are not recommended, since in the long term the success rate is poor.

Injuries not of Recent Origin. If the Class II injury is not of recent origin, the danger to the pulp from bacterial invasion via the dentinal tubules and to a lesser extent from thermal irritation, is considerable. In the immature tooth every effort should be made to maintain vitality, and although pulpotomy is best carried out as soon as possible it is not contra-indicated even several weeks after injury (Stewart, 1964). When treatment has been delayed in the mature tooth with a Class II injury, extirpation of the pulp is the treatment of choice.

Immediate Treatment Class III Injuries

Class III injuries include all degrees of pulpal exposure. As with Class I and Class II injuries, it is essential to carry out a thorough clinical and radiographic examination. When the classification has been established and soft tissue injuries and any displacements treated, the decision on procedure depends primarily on the stage of root development and may, therefore, be considered under two headings:

1. Treatment of the vital exposed pulp in an immature tooth with open apex.
2. Treatment of the vital exposed pulp in a mature tooth with closed apex.

Treatment of the non-vital tooth is not considered under the heading 'emergency treatment' and is dealt with in Chapter 5.

The Vital Tooth—Open Apex. The objective in treating the immature tooth with a Class III injury is to preserve the vitality of the pulp so that root development may proceed to apical closure, when the pulp can then be extirpated to facilitate the placement of a permanent restoration. The treatment which affords the most favourable prognosis is immediate pulpotomy. This is fully described in Chapter 5.

The operation of pulpotomy requires full patient co-operation and it follows that a shocked, apprehensive or frightened child, may not prove to be a suitable subject. It is permissible to defer pulp treatment for 24 to 48 hours. However, a sedative dressing placed without pressure should be applied before dismissing the patient. A new appointment should be arranged and premedication prescribed if thought necessary. In some cases it may be possible to carry out pulpotomy only under a general anaesthetic.

The Vital Tooth—Closed Apex. The Class III injury in the vital tooth with closed apex is best treated by immediate extirpation of the pulp. Any attempt to preserve the vitality of the pulp by less radical treatment is not recommended, since the exposed pulp, however minimal the exposure, must be regarded as contaminated and the prognosis therefore poor.

Immediate Treatment Class IV Injuries

Class IV injuries are those involving fracture of the root with or without fracture of the crown, with or without displacement of the tooth. The management of such cases depends primarily on the level of the root fracture as determined by radiographic examination.

Fracture of Coronal Third of Root. The characteristic clinical feature of coronal third fracture is excessive mobility of the coronal fragment. Because such fractures usually expose the pulp to contamination from the mouth and since the coronal fragment can rarely be satisfactorily retained, the immediate treatment is to remove the crown. If the fracture line is seen to extend more than 4 mm. below the gingival attachment in an oblique fracture, or is below the level of the alveolar crest in a transverse fracture, then the root should be extracted. A tooth with a short root, unsuitable for supporting a restoration, should also be extracted.

If a decision is made to retain the root, then immediate vital extirpation should be carried out with a view to sealing the apical 3 mm. either at the same visit or at a later appointment. To prevent encroachment of the gingivae on the root surface a zinc oxide/eugenol/cotton-wool pack should be placed in position before dismissing the patient. If time permits, at the emergency appointment a temporary post-retained acrylic crown will more adequately restrain the gingival tissues and also improve appearance.

Fracture of the Middle Third of the Root. Some mobility of the crown is a feature of middle third fractures and provided there has been no displacement of the coronal fragment the prognosis for retained pulpal vitality is good. In these circumstances treatment consists of immobilisation of the tooth by splinting as previously described.

In cases with coronal displacement immediate reduction, endodontic treatment and immobilisation are required for a favourable prognosis. The use of a Sved type of removable splint in these latter cases will permit the fitting of rubber dam during endodontic procedures.

Fracture of Apical Third of the Root. No immediate treatment is normally required for apical third fractures. They should, however, be kept under observation for possible loss of pulpal vitality.

REFERENCES

BARRIE, W. J. M. & HARGREAVES, J. A. (1969). Stainless steel crowns in children's dentistry. *Dent. News, Lond.* 6 No. 6, 8.

BENNETT, T. G. (1968). Replantation of teeth after trauma. *Med. Gaz., Newcastle*, 63, 30.

ELLIS, R. G. (1960). *The Classification and Treatment of Injuries to the Teeth of Children*, 4th ed. Chicago: Year Book Publishers.

FLANAGAN, V. D. & MYERS, H. I. (1958). Delayed reimplantation of second molars in the Syrian hamster. *Oral Surg.* 11, 1179.

HENNING, F. R. (1965). Reimplantation of luxated teeth. *Aust. dent. J.* 10, 306.

HORSNELL, A. M. & BROWN, G. (1956). Immediate splints for cases of trauma to the incisor teeth. *Dent. Practnr. dent. Rec.* 6, 148.

LÖE, H. & WAERHAUG, J. (1961). Experimental replantation of teeth in dogs and monkeys. *Archs oral Biol.* 3, 176.

SLACK, G. L. & BIRCH, R. H. (1958). Emergency treatment of dislodged incisors using soft alloy splints. *Dent. Practnr. dent. Rec.* 9, 74.

STEWART, D. J. (1964). Delayed pulpotomy in traumatized teeth: some further observations. *Dent. Practnr. dent. Rec.* 15, 58.

CHAPTER 5

Pulp Therapy

A BLOW on an anterior tooth may produce pulp damage in one or more of three ways: by traumatising the apical blood vessels it endangers the vitality of the whole pulp; by the production of a 'shock wave' effect in the pulp tissue it may disrupt the smaller blood vessels in the coronal pulp with associated haemorrhages and areas of necrosis; and finally by causing crown fracture it may expose the pulp.

Some degree of apical damage must occur in every injury. It is unfortunate that the extent of this damage cannot be as readily assessed as can fracture of the hard tissues of the tooth or its supporting structures, but instead must be deduced from radiographic and clinical examination with appropriate follow-up and an awareness of the probabilities in each type of injury.

The 'shock wave' effect is produced by momentary impaction of the tooth into its socket, particularly where the apex is incomplete. It is presumably a sudden sharp rise in intrapulpal pressure arising from this shock which produces rupture of the smaller blood vessels with subsequent haemorrhages. Where haemorrhage has been severe the crown shows discoloration and darkening.

Crown fracture is the most easily recognised result of trauma. If the fragment lost is not large, as in the Class I or Class II group, the only treatment required is protection of the exposed dentine and splinting of any slightly loosened tooth.

In the absence of displacement it is impossible to assess the extent of pulp damage. Vitality tests carried out shortly after trauma may provide little useful information. Teeth which fail to respond over the first few weeks are assumed to be in a state of shock, but when this phase passes a reaction to electric or thermal stimuli may return. During the waiting period a watch must be kept for any signs of deterioration of the pulp condition which would point to the need for immediate endodontic treatment.

Exposure or near exposure of the pulp as a result of fracture is dealt with by either pulpotomy or pulpectomy. Pulp capping as a clinical procedure has very limited application in all but the most favourable cases, and its use cannot be too strongly condemned in those pulps which are not only exposed but also otherwise injured.

While fracture of the root inevitably involves the pulp, the net result is usually favourable provided that the coronal pulp is not exposed. A large part of the energy of the blow is absorbed in the disruption of hard tissue with less damage to the apical vessels as a result. Decompression of the injured pulp seems to assist in pulp survival, and as long as the fracture is placed far enough apically to leave an adequate attachment between the coronal fragment and alveolar bone, the prognosis is good.

For ease of description the appropriate pulp therapy for each of five specific clinical categories is considered under the following headings:

1. The vital tooth with open apex.
2. The vital tooth with closed apex.
3. The non-vital tooth with open apex.
4. The non-vital tooth with closed apex.
5. Root fracture.

THE VITAL TOOTH WITH OPEN APEX

In the immature tooth pulp death is unlikely to arise from damage to the pulpal vessels passing through the wide apical opening. Any negative response to vitality tests carried out shortly after injury can be attributed to post-traumatic shock, and the return of normal sensation during the subsequent 2 to 6 weeks awaited with some confidence.

Disruption of the hard tissues is treated on the basis of the classification already given. Class I fractures require no further attention than the removal of sharp enamel edges. The management of Class II fractures depends on two factors—the remaining thickness of dentine between fracture surface and pulp, and the time that this surface has been left exposed to the oral environment without protection. Both these factors have a bearing on the possibility of bacterial penetration of the remaining dentine, and such invasion, combined with areas of haemorrhage in the coronal pulp, has a disastrous effect on the chances of pulp survival. No risks can be taken and all but the smallest of dentine exposures are covered as soon as possible with a zinc-oxide eugenol or calcium hydroxide layer. Where a few days or even weeks have elapsed since the injury, this form of cover may be used, but if there is any suspicion of reduced vitality or of increasing discoloration produced by extensive pulpal haemorrhage, then the case is regarded as falling into the same treatment category as the Class III fracture with pulp exposure.

Capping of an exposed pulp even if the exposure is small, the injury recent and the apex wide open, is to be avoided. While some pulps may respond favourably, the majority do not, and in the absence of any reliable guides to forming a prognosis, there is considerable danger of the condition of the capped pulp deteriorating into the most difficult case of all to treat, namely the non-vital tooth with open apex in a young and perhaps unco-operative child.

Because of the wide connection between pulp and periapical tissues of the immature tooth, the recovery powers of the young pulp are extremely good. When a Class III fracture with exposure has occurred the still vital pulp tissue forms for a short time an effective barrier to deeper bacterial invasion. The opportunity this presents must be grasped quickly. Early removal of damaged and contaminated tissue permits establishment of the line of pulp section at the cervical level of the tooth, providing a sterile wound placed in a relatively undamaged zone, and at the same time avoids the problem of treating and filling a root canal with apically diverging walls.

Although immediate pulpotomy is desirable, it should still be considered as a form of therapy even a week or two after injury. While the apex remains wide open the pulp is not to be regarded as a separate 'organ' which either lives or dies completely as it tends to do in the adult tooth. The excellent vascular supply permits the natural establishment of a 'line of resistance' within the pulp, and although such a state of affairs is temporary, it is worth exploring the neglected exposed pulp in the hope of establishing a healthy wound short of the apical opening and the apical formative tissue.

While delay in treating an exposed pulp may be due to neglect on the part of the child's parents, it may be the choice of the operator. A terrified child is not a suitable subject for pulpotomy, and these injuries do not present at the most convenient times in a busy practice. It is much better to place a temporary cover on the exposure and dismiss the patient with an appointment to return in 24 to 48 hours, premedicated if necessary.

If the child is very apprehensive, arrangements can be made to carry out the pulpotomy at the second visit under general anaesthesia.

Pulpotomy

After obtaining surface anaesthesia, local anaesthetic is administered using a fine-gauge needle. The traumatised tooth and its immediate neighbours are thoroughly cleaned with bristle brush and polishing paste to remove food debris and plaque.

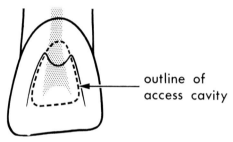

outline of access cavity

FIG. 77
Palatal opening for access to pulp chamber.

The more co-operative patients may accept rubber dam, but if the placement of a clamp or ligature on a tooth with no retentive undercuts is impossible or difficult, cotton rolls and an efficient saliva ejector should be used. A good chairside assistant will ensure that the saliva ejector is not removed by the child.

Access to the pulp is gained by carrying a small round bur (a No. 1 or No. 2) through the lingual surface at a level just incisal to the normally formed cingulum. If the crown fracture is large, straight-line access may be gained by plunging through the exposed dentine and along the tooth axis. The opening is enlarged and where necessary properly aligned with tapered fissure burs until its outline encompasses the underlying pulp chamber (Fig. 77). The fissure bur is never used to deepen the cavity, only to extend it by careful planing of the margins, otherwise a shelf may be formed and further exploration made difficult. Dentine debris is removed and haemorrhage is controlled by repeated irrigation with local anaesthetic solution, sterile saline or sterile water and the cavity dried by gentle application of sterile pledgets of cotton.

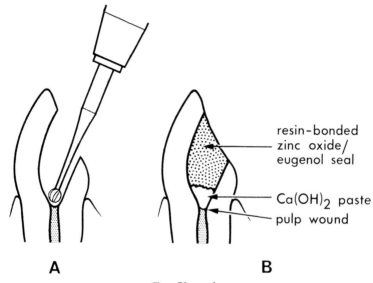

resin-bonded zinc oxide/ eugenol seal

Ca(OH)$_2$ paste

pulp wound

A   **B**

FIG. 78A and B

A section at level of cervical constriction; B dressing of pulp wound and sealing of cavity.

Views vary as to the best instrument for the removal of the coronal pulp, but the spoon excavator or bur used must be both sterile and sharp. Section is made at the level of the cervical constriction between coronal and radicular pulp so that the wound surface may be as small as possible (Fig. 78A). After further irrigation and gentle drying to permit a careful check and control haemorrhage, a 2 to 3 mm. layer of a non-setting calcium hydroxide paste is placed over the exposed tissue and the cavity filled with a resin bonded zinc oxide/eugenol cement (Fig. 78B). No pressure is placed on the pulp and the surface of the dressing is carefully kept out of occlusion. The parents are instructed to bring the child back in 6 to 8 weeks unless discomfort is experienced.

After 6 to 8 weeks a periapical radiograph will reveal, in successful cases, the presence of a calcified barrier beneath the original wound surface (Fig. 79A and B). If the barrier appears to be incomplete, then in the absence of symptoms the child should be dismissed for a further 4 weeks.

When radiographic evidence of a barrier is obtained, the tooth is isolated as before and the dressing removed. At this point the use of non-setting calcium hydroxide beneath the zinc oxide will be appreciated, as the cavity base is easily cleaned up without danger of damage. Usually a layer of dark, dried

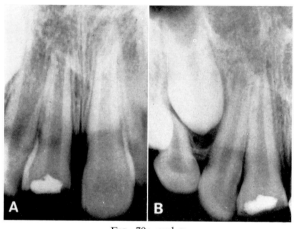

FIG. 79A and B

A radiograph showing pulpotomy of immature right central incisor; B radiograph, same tooth eighteen months later, note calcific barrier and apical closure.

blood is found immediately beneath the calcium hydroxide and this is gently scraped away with small excavators and probes to reveal a hard layer of dentine-like tissue beneath. This layer is in turn gently probed to detect any breaches which may exist.

Vitality of the remaining pulp may be determined by using cold air, cold water or even ethyl chloride on cotton against the barrier. The response is often weak, but this is related to the thickness of the barrier and to the fact that the radicular pulp has fewer nerve endings than the coronal pulp. In the presence of vitality and a complete barrier, consideration can be given to the form of the intermediate restoration (Fig. 80). In the following years root formation will continue and a normal apical constriction form. At about 16 years a full vital extirpation may be performed and a well-retained aesthetic post-core crown constructed. Views vary widely on the long-term success of pulpotomy, but where the problems of retention of an aesthetic restoration demand it, pulpectomy is normally carried out from 16 years onwards.

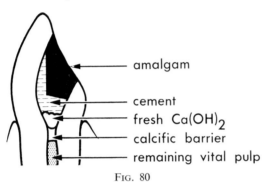

amalgam

cement

fresh $Ca(OH)_2$

calcific barrier

remaining vital pulp

FIG. 80

Intermediate restoration following pulpotomy.

The great advantages of pulpotomy in spite of the doubts on its long-term success are the one-visit control of a tooth which, when immature, presents a considerable endodontic problem, and the postponement of further and more arduous treatment to an age when the patient is more co-operative.

VITAL TOOTH WITH CLOSED APEX

It is practically impossible in a traumatised, fully formed tooth to establish the extent of pulp damage shortly after injury. Vitality tests are often negative, but this does not necessarily indicate pulp death, as sensitivity frequently returns in the ensuing days or weeks. Nor is the absence of crown fracture always a favourable sign. It may mean either that the blow has been a very mild one, or that the energy of a severe blow has been dissipated in other directions. Where the force has been applied along the long axis of the tooth, the tooth virtually becomes a missile driven into its own socket, and the force is transferred to the supporting tissues, particularly in the region of the apical periodontal membrane with severe damage to the vascular supply of the tooth, either by crushing or, where displacement occurs, by severing the vessels. A more obliquely aligned blow may produce crown or root fracture, usually with less damage to the apical vessels and a much better pulp prognosis.

In the absence of any of these obvious signs of pulp damage, the traumatised mature tooth is treated conservatively. Class I and Class II fractures are dealt with by grinding or the placement of protective dressings as already described and the tooth observed for a period of up to 6 weeks. If within this period the tooth shows a returning response to vitality tests, all may be well and intermediate restorative treatment begun. Further vitality tests should be carried out periodically in the ensuing year and subsequently at routine dental examinations. If there is no response at the end of the waiting period, the pulp may be presumed non-vital and immediate endodontic treatment carried out.

Discoloration is a common feature after trauma, and there is a danger in attaching too much significance to its presence. The colour change, initially to a red-pink shade, is an indication of pulpal haemorrhage and not of pulp death. Where the vascular supply is otherwise unimpaired and any crown fracture immediately sealed off from external irritation, breakdown and absorption of the extravasated haemoglobin follows with normal repair. The process of haemoglobin breakdown produces colour changes in the tooth similar to those seen in a bruise of the skin. Within a day or two the colour changes to a varying depth of blue-grey, which after about 2 weeks begins to fade to a permanent greyish tint. Failure of the colour to disappear completely is due to haemorrhage into the dentinal tubules followed by haemoglobin breakdown, without the possibility of final absorption of the coloured haemosiderin deposits.

Immediate pulp extirpation is indicated if the pulp has been exposed by crown fracture, or if a dentinal fracture runs very close to a pulp horn without actual exposure. Neither capping nor pulpotomy should be considered. If doubt remains as to how near the pulp is to exposure, the factors which will decide the appropriate treatment are the time since injury that the dentine has remained unprotected and the problem of later

placing a well-retained restoration without using the root canal.
It is a pointless exercise to conserve a pulp and then realise that
there is inadequate tissue left to carry a jacket crown.

When extirpation has been decided upon, it should be done
quickly, on the grounds that it is much simpler to carry out a
vital extirpation than to deal with a putrescent pulp and developing periapical reaction.

The procedure is quite standard and is well dealt with in
endodontic textbooks. Some points relevant to the management of incisors in the 9- to 10-year-old are worth mentioning.
Rubber dam application is desirable but may be difficult purely
because of lack of cervical undercut to retain a rubber dam
clamp or ligature. This difficulty can be overcome by shaping

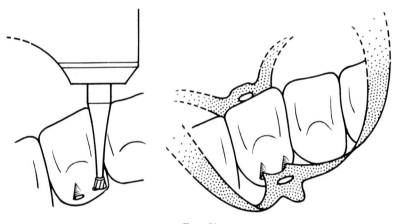

FIG. 81

Preparation of ledge to facilitate placement of rubber dam clamp.

the jaws of the chosen clamp with small carborundum stones
until it fits the tooth more closely. If the lack of an appropriate
inclined plane still prevents clamp placement, a small ledge may
be cut on the palatal surface of the tooth to provide the necessary 'foothold' for the beaks of the clamp (Fig. 81).

Entry to the pulp is made in the same way as for pulpotomy,
but the cervical constriction of the pulp canal, instead of being
left, is planed away with a tapered fissure but, preferably with
the end rounded, so as to provide a funnel-shaped opening
directly into and in line with the root canal.

Pulp extirpation using a single rotating barbed broach is often unsuccessful, especially where haemorrhage has rendered some areas of the tissue more friable. Removal of the pulp in one piece is more readily achieved if a second barbed broach is gently carried alongside the first and the handles then given a turn around each other so that the tissue is engaged in a sort of pincer movement (Fig. 82). This use of the two broaches is quite safe in the very wide canal of the young incisor.

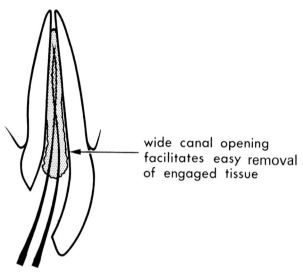

wide canal opening facilitates easy removal of engaged tissue

FIG. 82

Removal of pulp employing two barbed broaches.

Reaming is likely to be fruitless in the young tooth because of the canal width. Instead, more attention is paid to filing the canal walls to develop a smooth dentine surface.

Filing can be a dangerous procedure in inexpert hands, especially where the root appears to be completely formed but where in fact no proper apical constriction is present. A vigorous pumping action with no regard for accuracy of length can only lead to disaster. A good diagnostic radiograph with a measured radio-opaque point in position is taken after pulp removal and the tooth length calculated. One millimetre is subtracted from the total tooth length and this final figure noted as the 'working length'. Stops are placed to this length on all files used and great care taken to ensure that the file is placed no further up the canal than the stop at any time. Lateral force is applied only on withdrawal of the file and in this way the danger of producing an apical wound, churned up and choked with debris, is avoided. Thorough irrigation with a 1 per cent sodium hypochlorite solution alternating with sterile water is an essential adjunct to efficient root canal preparation. Root canal instruments cut more effectively in a wet field and debris is more easily moved from the canal without either apical penetration or impaction when repeated irrigation is maintained.

The choice of root filling techniques is varied, but the simplest ones rely on the selection of the widest gutta-percha point which will reach to the full working length, that is to the apical constriction. The first point chosen, if it appears to fill the canal reasonably well throughout its whole length, may be carried into place after gently spinning the selected root canal sealer up the dried canal on a lentulo spiral. If the fit is only good apically, it is wiser to resort to the multiple-point lateral condensation method, using the appropriate Kerr's spreaders to create space for additional gutta-percha points after the first one is in place. When the spreader can no longer be pushed into the canal, root filling is complete.

A final radiograph is taken to check the adequacy of the root filling. This should be dense, free from voids, extend to 0·5 to 1 mm. from the radiographic apex, and should at all points appear to be in close contact with the walls of the canal.

NON-VITAL TOOTH WITH OPEN APEX

Loss of vitality in the immature tooth is less the result of trauma alone than the product of pulpal damage and bacterial invasion, and these cases are usually the result of neglect of either Class III fractures or Class II fractures where the remaining dentine thickness alone has been inadequate to prevent bacterial penetration. The latter case is particularly unfortunate if the sensitivity of the exposed dentine has not been enough to drive an apprehensive child to seek treatment, and indeed delay often improves the situation as far as the patient is concerned by allowing the onset of pulp necrosis.

When necrosis has occurred and radiographs show an associated area of apical rarefaction, treatment is urgent, because in spite of radiographic appearances the formative region may not yet be irreparably damaged and early endodontic therapy may still allow root completion.

Rubber dam is applied only on a very co-operative patient and on a tooth which has erupted enough to retain a clamp or ligature. On no account should a young child's limited tolerance be exhausted by rubber dam placement.

The access cavity must be large enough to encompass the large underlying pulp and also to allow access of root canal files to the diverging walls of the apical half of the canal. When prepared, the cavity is cleared of dentine debris and any superficial gangrenous pulp tissue is removed with a sharp sterile excavator. The cavity is gently swabbed with a mild antiseptic solution (e.g. 0·05 per cent hibitane) in cotton, dried and one or two drops of root canal medicament (e.g. camphorated monochlorphenol or CHAMP) applied to the pulp surface.

The remaining pulp debris is gently removed on barbed broaches carried to a length calculated from the preliminary radiograph. This length can only be an approximation, but to avoid unnecessary penetration of the apical opening should err on the short side.

Depending on the position of the line of demarcation of vital and non-vital tissue, haemorrhage may be a problem, but it can be controlled by repeated irrigation with either local anaesthetic containing a vasoconstrictor, saturated calcium hydroxide solution, or even sterile water. Haemorrhage is not controlled by continually disturbing a wound surface with paper points. If local anaesthetic solution is used, the effluent should be collected on cotton rolls because of its unpleasant taste.

On account of the lack of the 'stop' effect of an apical constriction in the immature tooth, careful estimation of length and the use of instrument markers is essential. A narrow diagnostic wire in the very wide canal can give rise to considerable error in length estimation due to a difference of angulation between tooth and wire. To avoid such error, as wide a gutta-percha point as will sit comfortably in the canal is used. It is cut off level with the incisal edge, removed, measured, and replaced in its original position. A radiograph is taken and the length calculated in the usual way.

Neither the shape nor the diameter of the canal makes it suitable for reaming and only files can effectively plane and smooth the canal walls, but they must be used with great care because the dentine at the forming root end is very thin and damage to this region will destroy any chance of subsequent root formation. Stops are used on all files to a level 2 mm. short of the estimated length and filing carried out, with a more gentle pull movement than in the fully formed tooth. The entire circumference of the canal is covered in this way. Dentine shavings, debris and exudate are thoroughly washed out by repeated irrigation and the canal dried with sterile cotton and paper points. The apically diverging walls of a 'blunderbuss' canal can only be reached where the access cavity is wide enough to allow the file to lie obliquely across the canal. A little may be added to the instrument length to compensate for the altered position, but so great is the danger of unnecessarily traumatising the formative area of the tooth and the apical wound tissue, that such filing is kept to a minimum, and reliance for the re-moval of necrotic debris placed mainly on the prolonged use of a warm irrigant and tissue solvent such as sodium hypochlorite (1 per cent solution).

Root filling is generally an unsatisfactory procedure in the immature tooth with wide-open apex when any of the conven-tional techniques are used. Apart from the shape of the canal, it is often extremely difficult to keep it clear enough of serous exudate to allow good adaptation between sealer and dentine. While condensation techniques may be used in the parallel-sided canal, proper condensation is difficult and in the 'blunderbuss' canal virtually impossible.

Three main trends have been developed in dealing with the problem of filling the root canal of the partly formed tooth. The first, which ensures a good apical seal, involves the placement of a conventional root filling followed by apicectomy.

Unfortunately such treatment precludes the possibility of further root development and also leaves a tooth which is diffi-cult to restore later with a post retained crown. If the problem of apicectomy in the young child is added to these disadvantages,

F

the general preference for other methods can be readily understood.

The second approach has been to use non-setting dressings
containing iodoform or antibiotic pastes as temporary fillings
after preliminary canal cleansing. Accuracy of fit is not necessary and in the event of periodontitis giving rise to discomfort,
the dressing is easily removed and drainage established. At a
later stage, if root formation proceeds to completion, a conventional root canal filling may be placed. If root growth is
arrested by apical destruction, root filling and apicectomy are
necessary, but the temporary filling may gain a few valuable
years for the operator, by which time the apicectomy can be
carried out simply under local anaesthesia.

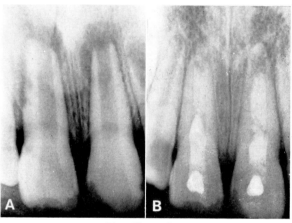

Fig. 83A and B
A radiograph of non-vital immature central incisor teeth;
B radiograph same teeth, showing calcified apical barrier.

The third method (Kennedy, 1967) overcomes most of the
problems, not only of root filling, but of canal preparation
in the tooth with open apex. After mechanical preparation of
the canal walls with root canal files accompanied by frequent
irrigation, the prepared canal is dried and a calcium hydroxide
water paste spun into place using an engine driven lentulo spiral,
and sealed with a thick layer of resin bonded zinc oxide/eugenol
cement. After 12 weeks the tooth is isolated and both the seal
and the calcium hydroxide removed. The presence of a clinical
barrier which can be percussed (Fig. 83A and B) indicates a

successful result and the root canal is filled in any of the conventional ways with little danger of overfilling. In the absence
of a barrier at 12 weeks the dressing may be repeated, and
a successful case is reported at 32 weeks (Kennedy, 1967).
Results using this technique in the young patient are excellent
and continued root formation appears to be unimpaired by the
use of calcium hydroxide pastes.

Non-vital Tooth with Closed Apex

Pulp death is assumed in a fully formed traumatised anterior
tooth if there is no response to stimulation 6 weeks after injury.
Even after this period the cases which gave a vital response
must be observed over a period of several months to detect
any post-traumatic deterioration of the pulp. If such careful
checks are carried out, pulp extirpation when necessary may be
performed before the development of symptoms or apical
pathology and in some instances before total pulp necrosis has
occurred.

Such a carefully observed case may be treated exactly as a
vital extirpation, but unfortunately the very absence of symptoms or other signs of deterioration often leads the patient and
even the operator to a false sense of security. A necrotic
untreated pulp produces, by autolysis, irritation of the periapical
tissues and this may be severe enough to produce a reaction in
the form of a periapical granuloma or chronic apical abscess,
either of which is eventually discovered by either routine radiography or vitality tests.

Bacterial invasion of a necrotic pulp is an ever-present danger.
The entry may be by way of defects in the crown, by extension
from gingival lesions which share a common lymph drainage
with the pulp, or by anachoresis. Such contamination may
produce a violent tissue reaction (for example an acute periapical abscess) with severe pain and marked swelling due in the
first instance to oedema and later, if untreated, to oedema
combined with pus formation. The patient is extremely uncom-
fortable, and the tooth usually exquisitely tender to touch.
Swelling may involve the lip and cheek as far as the orbit when
an upper tooth is involved or the inferior border of the mandible
and associated submental and submandibular regions if a lower

incisor is involved. A tense swelling may be observed in the vestibule and the involved tooth is mobile, often alarmingly so, and usually slightly extruded.

Initial treatment should be kept to the minimum required to relieve pain. Early swellings are usually mainly oedematous and little is gained by incision, but once the vestibular swelling, or in the case of the upper lateral, palatal swelling, shows signs of being fluctuant, incision followed by expansion with artery forceps down to the bone will produce a flow of pus and immediate relief. An H-shaped piece of rubber dam inserted into the incision maintains drainage for several days. Whether or not incision is necessary, drainage must in all cases be established by opening into the pulp chamber. The extremely tender tooth is supported firmly on its labial side by the operator's fingers and entry made against this resistance by gently applying an air-rotor to the palatal surface. There is no need at this stage to do any more than provide access to carry a barbed broach far enough up the canal to clear any pulp debris or pus. The canal may be irrigated with a warm solution of either sterile saline or sterile water and is then left for 48 to 72 hours to drain and to allow inflammation to settle. The child's parents are warned to return if the pain has not subsided within a few hours. Resolution is assisted by regular use of warm mouthwashes.

Where the patient has an elevated temperature and is obviously unwell, an antibiotic should be prescribed to assist recovery.

At the second visit the patient's condition presents a completely changed picture. The pain should have disappeared entirely and the swelling be much less. Any food debris in the pulp chamber is teased out with a barbed broach and the chamber irrigated with sterile saline or water. The canal is explored to an estimated length with a barbed broach, after which the loosened contents are washed out. A measured length of wire is placed in the root canal and a periapical radiograph taken. Thus the exact tooth length may now be calculated.

At this point a decision is made whether to proceed further at this visit. If there is still slight discomfort and some pus or exudate coming from the periapical region, nothing more should be done than to place a pledget of cotton loosely in the pulp chamber and arrange for another visit in 48 to 72 hours.

If the canal is fairly clean and the tooth symptomless, mechanical preparation may be begun at the second visit. For the older child rubber dam should be applied as routine. Reaming and filing are carried out as for a vital extirpation. All instruments used in the canal must carry stops to prevent trauma to the tissue beyond the apical constriction, and the canal is repeatedly flushed with irrigants during instrumentation to avoid forcing debris through into the periapical tissues. Each time a reamer or file is removed from the canal, the debris between its blades must be wiped off in an antiseptic solution (e.g. 0·05 per cent hibitane) before it may be replaced, otherwise a 'build up' of debris will occur and the normal spiral outward movement of dentine chips and debris prevented.

At subsequent visits, after irrigation and drying, a root canal medicament is carried into the canal on a short section of paper point or on a cotton pledget and sealed in with resin bonded zinc oxide/eugenol cement. The medicaments of choice are camphorated monochlorphenol, beechwood creosote, cresatin, CHAMP (Atkinson and Hampson, 1964) and many others. All are used sparingly and the medicaments changed at each visit.

When the tooth is symptomless and the canal dry and clear of exudate, it may be considered ready for root filling. Bacteriological examinations may be carried out, but their accuracy and value are very much in doubt.

If the crown of the tooth is badly discoloured or damaged, it may be scheduled for replacement with a post-core retained porcelain jacket crown when the root filling is complete. To avoid unnecessary work only the apical third of the root canal need be filled, leaving the coronal two-thirds ready for crown preparation. A single cone is selected as before, but after the sealer has been spun into the canal the apical 4 or 5 mm. of the cone is cut off and tagged on to the warm tip of a root canal spreader. The stop on the spreader is adjusted so that the length from the tip of the short gutta-percha point to the stop equals the total 'working length' of the tooth. The point is lightly smeared with root canal sealer and carried into place until the stop is level with the incisal edge. The spreader is twisted free of the point and removed. The final position of the apical third filling is checked by carrying the remainder of the initially selected gutta-percha point up the canal, when it should butt on to the apical third as the original 'working length' mark reaches the incisal edge. Finally, cotton-wool is placed loosely in the canal and a temporary seal inserted until crown construction at a later date.

Other acceptable root filling techniques include the use of apical third silver points. The selected point is almost severed at a chosen distance (3 to 4 mm.) from the tip with a pair of wire cutters and the apical portion coated with a creamy mix of root canal sealer. The point is carried firmly up the root canal to the measured length with pliers and the main part of the point removed by twisting it free of the apical third. Perhaps the main disadvantage of this technique is that in the event of failure of the endodontic treatment at a later date, removal of the apical third silver point, other than by apicectomy, is virtually impossible.

There seems to be little indication for the use of silver points for full-length root canal filling in the young incisor, particularly in view of the difficulty of part removal at a later date if a post-retained crown is envisaged. Narrow and curved canals, which are the usual indications for the use of full silver points, seldom occur in the anterior teeth of children.

Root Fracture

The management of traumatised anterior teeth with root fracture depends mainly on whether the fracture involves the coronal, middle or apical third of the root.

Fracture of the Coronal Third of the Root

The most obvious feature of fracture at this level is excessive mobility of the crown. If the fracture line is transverse it cannot be seen other than by radiographic examination, but if it is oblique or transverse with an oblique component, it usually crosses the gingival attachment to expose the pulp to the mouth.

Because of the discomfort of the mobile fragment, these cases usually present very early. The normal investigation of all other possibly involved teeth is carried out in the usual way. Routine periapical radiographs, as well as giving information on other possible fractures, allow an accurate assessment of the extent

of the specific root fracture and the length of root remaining.
If the fracture line extends more than about 4 mm. below the
gingival attachment in an oblique fracture or if the tooth has a
short root, then extraction of the entire tooth is the wisest
course. Transverse fractures are more difficult to manage
than oblique ones by any of the methods mentioned later, and
extraction is usually carried out if the fracture is below the level
of the alveolar crest, as seen on radiographs.

A final decision on conservation cannot be reached until the
crown has been removed and the shape and depth of the fracture
examined. If the case is unsuitable, the root is removed immediately; otherwise, the case is prepared for vital pulp extirpation. Haemorrhage is controlled by papillary infiltration of
local anaesthetic containing a vasoconstrictor and packing with
epinephrine impregnated string (Gingi-pak*). The remaining
pulp is removed on barbed broaches and the canal prepared for
root filling in exactly the same way as for a conventional vital
extirpation. At the same visit, time permitting, the apical
portion of the canal is sealed with a 3 mm. gutta-percha point
and root canal sealer as previously described. If this is not
possible, a short medicated paper point is sealed in the root
canal for 48 to 72 hours. The root face is then covered with a
firm pack of zinc oxide/eugenol with included cotton strands
to prevent encroachment of the gingivae. If it has been possible
to place an apical third root filling at the first visit, a temporary
post-retained acrylic crown which restrains the gingival tissues
even more effectively may be used.

The main problem in constructing crowns for these cases lies
in the production of an accurate impression of the root face,
and one of several methods may be employed.

Ellis (1960) suggests the use of the natural crown as the restoration, so avoiding altogether the problem of taking an impression. The canal is prepared either with precision reamers or
tapered burs, and a post constructed from the corresponding
gauge post wire or from an accurate wax pattern. This is tried
in the canal and its projecting length adjusted until the previously hollowed-out crown can be seated over it and fitted
firmly on to the root surface (Fig. 84). When this has been
achieved, the post is cemented into the root canal. The crown

* Gingi-pak is distributed by Surgident Ltd., Los Angeles 66, California.

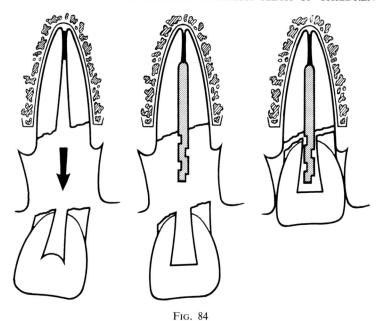

FIG. 84

Method of adapting natural crown following coronal third root fracture.

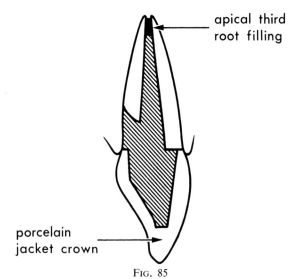

apical third
root filling

porcelain
jacket crown

FIG. 85

Post core crown replacing lost shoulder to
restore gingival level.

is filled with a suitable shade of crown cement and carried into place over the post and against the root surface.

A second method (Clyde, 1965) uses the fracture surface of the excised crown as the impression of the root and to this is added an impression of the root canal in greenstick composition. A model is cast and on this a post core is built up with the lost shoulder restored to gingival level (Fig. 85). When the cast

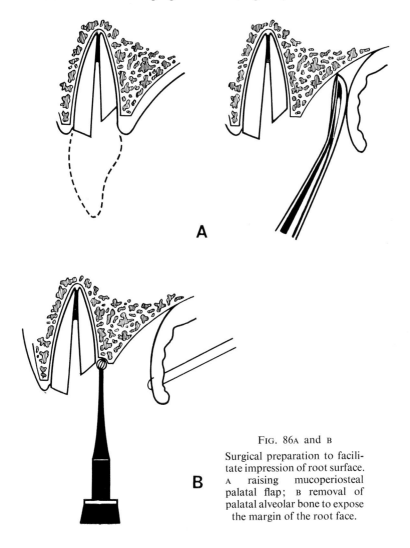

FIG. 86A and B

Surgical preparation to facilitate impression of root surface. A raising mucoperiosteal palatal flap; B removal of palatal alveolar bone to expose the margin of the root face.

post core is cemented the case is continued normally for a porcelain jacket crown. The method is usually only successful when the fracture surface is on two planes—transverse and oblique. During impression taking the oblique component guides the crown into place and the transverse component acts as a stop. In this way only may accurate seating be achieved.

The third method, useful when the crown cannot be used, involves a surgical approach. A mucoperiosteal flap is raised, either labially, or more commonly palatally, depending on the site of the deepest part of the fracture (Fig. 86A). Alveolar bone projecting beyond the root surface is cut back with a round bur until the tooth margins stand clear of bone (Fig. 86B). Any reshaping of the root surface, such as a reverse bevel on the root face for retention, is carried out and the root canal prepared with finishing burs.

The mucoperiosteal flap is held back, in the case of a palatal flap with sutures tied round the upper posterior teeth, the exposed area irrigated with sterile water and dried with sterile gauze packs.

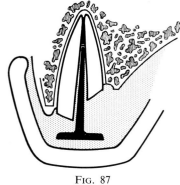

FIG. 87

Impression technique following surgical preparation.

Light-bodied rubber base is spun into the root canal, reinforced with a metal or plastic post and an overall tray impression in heavy bodied rubber base taken (Fig. 87). A stone die is cast in the laboratory and on this a post crown and veneer may be accurately constructed to the same design as in the previous method.

Fracture of the Middle Third of the Root

Fracture of the middle third of the root is often suspected because of crown mobility, but can only be distinguished from slight displacement by careful radiographic examination. Root fracture of the middle third is often accompanied by retained vitality, presumably because of the decompression effect of distraction of the opposing fracture surfaces on the pulp. In fact, it is common to find that of two traumatised central incisors one is apparently undamaged or only slightly damaged but non-vital while the other, showing root fracture, remains vital.

In the weeks following trauma there is resorption of cementum and dentine around the fracture surfaces, apparent on radiographs as a rounding off of the sharp fracture edges. Resorption usually ceases after the first few weeks and some degree of repair with cementoid-type tissue occurs. This has been reported as occasionally joining the two fragments (Cawson, 1968), but even in these cases the union is weak and is never a true repair such as that occurring after bone fracture. At best cementoid type tissue seals the resorbed dentine surfaces, and a shelf of alveolar bone may even form between the two fragments so that the coronal fragment is once again a normally supported, if abbreviated, tooth.

Treatment consists, where the pulp is vital and the coronal fragment fairly firm, of nothing more than immobilisation of the tooth by splinting for 3 months until periodontal inflammation has subsided and repair is well under way. After removal of the splint any occlusal interferences between the fractured tooth and its opponents are relieved, and periodic vitality tests carried out to ensure continuing pulp vitality.

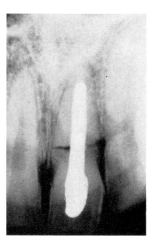

FIG. 88
Radiograph of endodontic splint.

If the coronal fragment has a root component so short and so mobile that long-term retention is unlikely, immediate vital pulp extirpation followed by the placement of a rigid root filling to splint the two parts together will give a satisfactory result for at least a number of years (Fig. 88). The same procedure is adopted where pulp death is recent. During endodontic treatment temporary splinting is achieved by the use of a removable acrylic plate of the Sved type, so that rubber dam may be placed. When the canal has been prepared a length of stainless-steel wire is ground to the appropriate taper, checked by radiography for length and fit and, when satisfactory, sealed in the root canal with the sealer of choice.

Middle third fractures which have not been treated shortly after trauma have a very poor prognosis. Internal splinting is virtually impossible because of the difficulty of finding the root

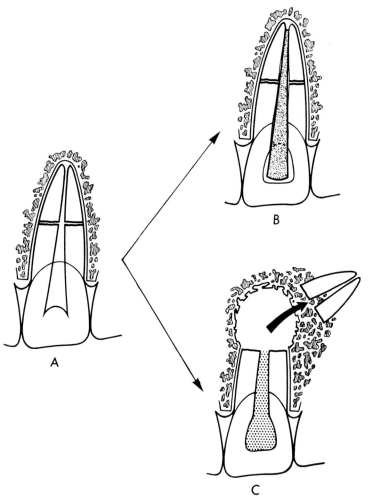

FIG. 89

Root filling and apicectomy, middle third root fracture. Alternative approaches to middle third root fracture (A) are either B,—endodontic splinting or C,—root filling to the fracture line and surgical removal of the apical fragment.

canal of the apical fragment with root canal instruments after resorption and repair have begun. If the coronal fragment is reasonably firm it may be root filled alone and the apical root excised together with any associated granulation tissue (Fig. 89), but in these circumstances the patient should be warned of the shortened life expectancy of the tooth as a result of physiological gingival recession and alveolar bone loss.

Fracture, especially of the middle third, may be associated with dislocation of the coronal fragment. The prognosis for such cases is not good unless reduction and endodontic treatment are performed immediately. Bacterial contamination is a hazard, and adequate retention of the crown for any length of time is unlikely unless endodontic splinting can be carried out.

Fracture of the Apical Third of the Root

Fracture of the apical third is not often seen in the incisors of children, but routine radiographs must be taken as mobility is not a feature of fracture in this region and these injuries may be easily overlooked. If vitality is retained, no treatment is required other than a watch for subsequent loss of vitality, or resorption. Where the pulp is necrotic, its early removal followed by root canal debridement and mechanical preparation to the level of the fracture is necessary. At the final visit the canal is root filled and the apical root fragment removed surgically.

Associated Crown Fracture and Root Fracture

Fortunately this combination is uncommon, but where it does occur in one tooth, a severe blow is usually the cause.

The Class I or mild Class II fracture may adversely affect the prognosis for a vital pulp when associated with root fracture, but the treatment is essentially that for the appropriate root fracture together with protection of any exposed dentine.

The greatest complication occurs when an extensive Class II or a Class III fracture accompanies root fracture.

Where the associated root fracture involves the coronal third of the root, treatment of the root fracture is altered only in so far as the use of the severed crown as the restoration (Ellis, 1960) becomes impracticable. The other methods outlined above are still applicable to these cases.

The fair prognosis for the pulp in a tooth with middle third fracture of the root can no longer be anticipated when associated with Class III or extensive Class II fracture. The usual treatment is that for recent middle third root fractures with a non-vital pulp, namely temporary splinting with a removable appliance, pulp extirpation and endodontic splinting. A porcelain veneer crown is constructed later, using the coronal dentine supported by the endodontic post as a core.

Retained pulp vitality is also unlikely in apical third fractures associated with Class III or extensive Class II fractures. Routine endodontic therapy and post-core construction for the major fragment produce a good result. If the extirpated pulp is vital, the apical fragment may be left, but in the presence of apical infection it is better that an apicectomy be performed. In these circumstances the approach may conveniently be modified by constructing the post core and porcelain veneer while the root canal is still unfilled, and only cementing the two parts in place immediately prior to apicectomy. In this way the maximum length of root canal can be used for post retention, and the post in fact provides the apical seal. The only precaution needed is to ensure that cementation of the crown and apicectomy are done at the same visit.

REFERENCES

ATKINSON, A. M. & HAMPSON, E. L. (1964). Sterilisation of root canals. *Br. dent. J.* **117**, 526.

CAWSON, R. A. (1968). *Essentials of Dental Surgery and Pathology*, 2nd ed. London: Churchill.

CLYDE, J. S. (1965). Transverse-oblique fractures of the crown with extension below the epithelial attachment. *Br. dent. J.* **119**, 402.

ELLIS, R. G. (1960). *The Classification and Treatment of Injuries to the Teeth of Children*, 4th ed. Chicago: Year Book Publishers.

KENNEDY, G. D. C., McLUNDIE, A. C. & DAY, R. M. (1967). Calcium hydroxide, its role in a simplified endodontic technique. *Dent. Mag. oral Top.* **84**, 51.

CHAPTER 6

Intermediate Treatment for Injured Incisor Teeth

FOLLOWING emergency measures to protect traumatised incisor teeth, the continued aim is to preserve the vitality of the pulp or to retain the root for crowning.

VITAL TEETH

An interim period exists between the recovery of a tooth from the immediate effects of injury and the time when a permanent restoration can be placed. These interim restorations are classed as semi-permanent. The main points affecting treatment of injured vital teeth in children are:

1. Dentinal tubules are wider and the cutting of young dentine with subsequent cementation of a fabricated crown may cause inflammatory changes resulting in pulpal death.
2. The pulp chamber in the crown of newly erupted teeth is large and it recedes with age as further dentine is laid down. A large pulp chamber is easily exposed in any extensive restorative procedure. Any preparation, therefore, undertaken on a newly erupted tooth should aim at removal of minimal tooth tissue which will be restored by a material strong in thin section.
3. The full length of the clinical crown of a newly erupted tooth is not established. Thus, satisfactory routine restorative procedures are difficult to achieve. The junction between a restoration and the contour of the gingival margin must be critically assessed and continually observed, as this junction will become visible as gingival recession proceeds.
4. The root continues to develop for 3 to 4 years after tooth eruption and every precaution must be taken to ensure that pulpal death does not occur before root formation is complete.

As the child becomes older, these differences become less marked and it is, therefore, not advisable to consider permanent crowning until the child has reached approximately 17 years of age when most developmental changes will have taken place.

Semi-permanent Restorations

Fractures which require semi-permanent restorations frequently have a diagonal fracture line from the incisal edge running towards the gingival margin (Fig. 90). The teeth most commonly fractured are maxillary central incisors and the restorative procedures described will refer to these teeth although the method would be the same for any incisor tooth.

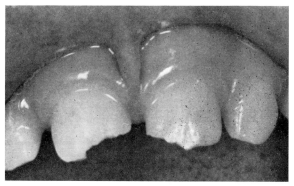

Fig. 90
Diagonal fractures of maxillary central incisor teeth.

Several crowns have been described for these interim restorations. In order to avoid the risk of pulpal exposure, preparations involving retention by cutting pin-holes, retention grooves or ledges into the dentine are best discarded. A horizontal fracture, however, can be safely restored using friction-grip pins. Markley pins (1958) are also permissible, but the pulp must be protected (Figs 91 and 92). However, two satisfactory types of preparation are available, which fulfil all the requirements for a semi-permanent restoration, namely the reverse retention crown and basket crown. The determining factor for the reverse retention crown is that at least half the crown length remains on the shortest proximal margin while the

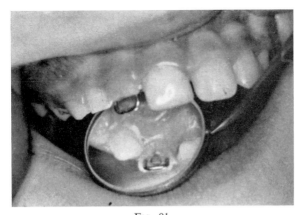

FIG. 91

Pinning a horizontal fracture of a maxillary central incisor.
Protection of the pulp is essential with calcium hydroxide or
a non-irritant cement, when pins are cemented.

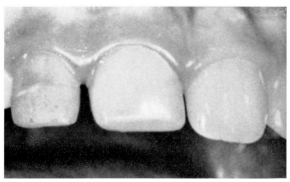

FIG. 92

Same tooth, shown in Figure 91, restored with acrylic.

basket crown is indicated when tooth loss is more severe
(Fig. 93).

In principle, both restorations are gold shoulderless veneer
crowns which cover the incisal edge, palatal and proximal
surfaces with a thin layer of gold. The two types differ only in
the way that retention is obtained against palatal displacement.
The reverse retention crown obtains retention against displacement by wrapping the proximal portions of gold on to the labial
surface; the basket crown achieves retention by an extension

G

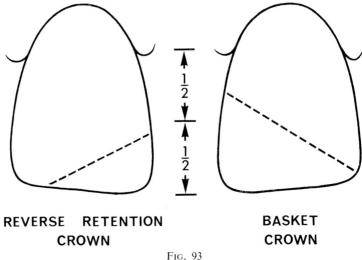

REVERSE   RETENTION   BASKET
         CROWN   CROWN

Fig. 93

Indications for reverse retention and basket crown restorations.

from its proximal edges at the cervical margin across the labial
face of the tooth (Fig. 94).

Tooth Assessment

A minimum period of 12 weeks should elapse between the
time of the fracture and the commencement of the preparation.
This allows the pulp to recover fully and for the operator to
determine whether vitality has been maintained.

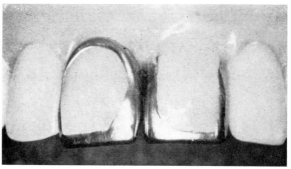

Fig. 94

Basket crown right maxillary central incisor and reverse
retention crown left centre incisor.

Before preparation the tooth should be symptom-free and show normal response to pulp testing. A periapical radiograph should be taken for later assessment in routine follow-up examinations. Study models to assess the alignment and the occlusion of the teeth are useful in planning the aesthetics and function of the restoration before commencing preparation. If the patient is young and apprehensive, the temporary crown can be left in place until the treatment is readily accepted.

Preparation

The first five stages are the same for both reverse retention and basket crowns and these will be detailed together, the different methods of retention for the two crowns will then be discussed individually.

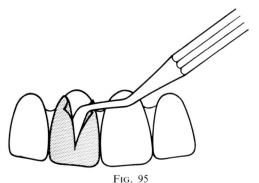

Fig. 95

Method for removing a temporary
stainless steel crown.

Local anaesthetic should be given and normal infiltration techniques for anterior tooth conservation are adequate.

The temporary crown should be gently removed with crown-removing pliers or by careful easing from the cervical margin with a large excavator. Other types of temporary protection can be removed in a similar way. If the crown is difficult to remove, this is best achieved by cutting a groove from the cervical margin with a fissure bur and splitting the crown open with a plastic instrument (Fig. 95). This method will always allow easy and gentle removal of a temporary crown (Barrie

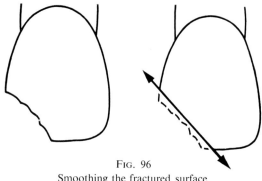

FIG. 96
Smoothing the fractured surface.

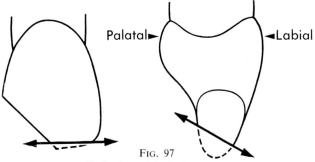

Palatal► ◄Labial

FIG. 97
Reduction of the incisal edge.

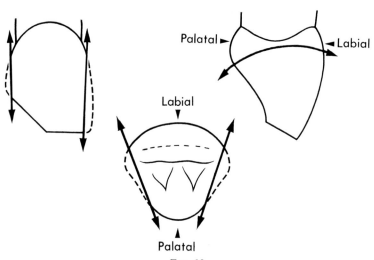

Palatal ► ◄ Labial

Labial
▼

Palatal
▲

FIG. 98
Preparation of proximal slices.

and Hargreaves, 1969). The preparation procedure is as follows:

1. The fracture surface is smoothed and straightened with a disc or stone (Fig. 96).
2. The clinical crown is reduced by approximately one-fifth of its length with a diamond or carborundum stone. Slightly more reduction is made on the palatal surface making a plane of approximately 45° to the long axis of the tooth (Fig. 97).
3. With a diamond or carborundum disc shoulderless slices are cut on the proximal surfaces. These slices converge slightly in a palatal direction and also towards the incisal edge (Fig. 98). This is best completed by placing the stationary disc at the crest of the gingival papilla and withdrawing in an incisal direction while cutting. This method avoids gingival trauma and eliminates the possibility of unwanted shoulders or undercuts. Should separation be needed to admit the disc, this can be obtained by use of a metal abrasive strip or separating disc.

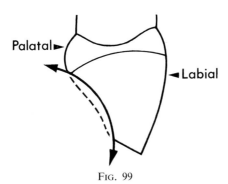

FIG. 99
Palatal reduction.

4. The next stage is reduction of the palatal surface. This involves minimal reduction to provide enough space for the palatal gold of the restoration without occlusal interference and further eliminates any grooves or fissures in the enamel. The reduction, which should not penetrate dentine in any part, permits a feather edge to be placed at

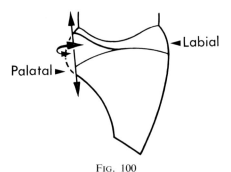

FIG. 100
Palatal smoothing at the cervical margin.

the gingival margin (Fig. 99). This can be readily completed with a small diamond wheel.
5. Further smoothing to obtain additional retention is made
   in the cervical area of the crown on the palatal aspect using
   a diamond fissure bur. A wall parallel with the long axis
   of the tooth is produced and this wall joins the proximal
   surfaces on the palatal aspect (Fig. 100).

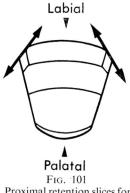

FIG. 101
Proximal retention slices for
a reverse retention crown.

6. At this stage the two preparations
   differ.
a. *Reverse Retention Crown.* Two
   small slices are made on the labial
   edge of the proximal slices, so
   angled that the preparation allows
   the restoration to be wrapped on to
   the labial surface. This is completed with a small diamond or
   carborundum disc. These extra
   slices converge towards the labial
   and prevent the restoration from
   being displaced palatally (Fig.
   101).

b. *Basket Crown.* Should the labial face of the tooth be so
   convex that an undercut exists on the long axis of the
   crown, it is necessary to remove some enamel with a
   diamond taper fissure bur (Fig. 102). The enamel is never
   removed to expose dentine.

These two steps—either 6a or 6b—complete the preparations.

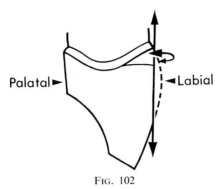

Palatal ► ◄ Labial

FIG. 102

Cervical smoothing on the labial surface, for
a basket crown.

Impression Techniques

The impression can be taken with impression compound or
rubber base material. For single crowns, greenstick impression
material is reliable, efficient and rapid. This method is detailed
with a 'carry-in' technique using greenstick material in a copper
ring. For this technique a ring is selected a size larger than
that which just fits the tooth. It is then annealed to remove any
inherent springiness which could cause distortion of the impression. The incisal rim is turned out to provide a work-hardened
margin to aid handling of the soft band. The ring must be
placed with a labial inclination to avoid undercuts made by
the curved labial surface of the tooth. The gingival periphery
of the ring is trimmed and smoothed to follow the outline of
the preparation. This fitting edge is then turned in to reduce
the diameter of the ring and provide a snug fit with the tooth
surface below the margin of the preparation (Fig. 103).

The gingival crevice will contain undercuts because of the
shape of the tooth, and should the ring pass too far below the
gingival margin, these undercuts will fill with impression compound causing distortion on removal. It is possible to control
the depth to which the copper band penetrates the gingival
crevice by the use of stops cut at each proximal side of the
incisal edge of the ring. The resultant tabs are turned out to
engage adjacent teeth and are stiffened with solder at the point
where they meet the ring. By this means, placing of the ring is

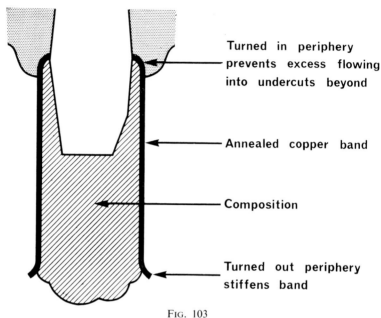

Turned in periphery prevents excess flowing into undercuts beyond

Annealed copper band

Composition

Turned out periphery stiffens band

FIG. 103
Diagram to show the fitting of a copper ring for impression taking.

controlled, unless undue force is used when seating (Fig. 104).

The sticks of greenstick are usually larger than the copper bands used. If this is the case, a stick of compound is warmed, reduced in diameter until it is a sliding fit within the ring and then allowed to cool. The greenstick is placed within the

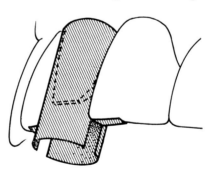

FIG. 104
Method of producing stiffened tabs for a
copper ring, to prevent placing the ring too
far gingivally.

ring and the end which contacts the tooth warmed in such a way that a hard core is left to act as a plunger.

The filled band is placed on to the tooth, using the finger-tips to press it home. The material in the ring is allowed to flow back, preventing a large collar of material flowing out at the gingival margin and obscuring the field. When the ring is fully home the plunger is pressed, forcing the greenstick material around the preparation.

One of the common faults with this type of impression is the use of too small a ring, which prevents adaption of impression compound whatever the pressure used. After 3 minutes under pressure to allow flow and cooling, the ring is removed. The path of removal should follow the labial inclination of the ring.

The preparation is now protected using the original temporary crown, and the patient is discharged. If the temporary crown had to be cut for removal, it may be necessary to fit a new crown.

Before the second visit, a transfer coping made of cold-cure acrylic resin is prepared on an accurate model.

At the second appointment the coping is fitted to the tooth. (Fig. 105). Because it is meant to be withdrawn in an overall impression, the coping should be grooved on its outer surfaces to provide retention and reduced on its proximal surfaces to allow the impression material to flow around the mesial and distal surfaces of the adjacent teeth. With the coping in place on the tooth an overall impression in alginate or rubber base is taken and the coping withdrawn in the impression material.

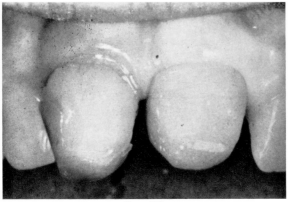

FIG. 105
Transfer copings in place on teeth.

The die is coated with petroleum jelly as a separating medium and is pushed home into the coping (Fig. 106). The model is now cast and when removed from the impression the die will be found in its correct position relative to the adjacent teeth. An impression of the opposite arch is taken, cast and the two models articulated.

The 'waxing up' procedure for the semi-permanent crowns is given in Appendix C and Appendix D.

The crown is cast in a platinised gold, which is stronger in thin section than the softer golds. After casting, the crown is polished on the copper die and, in the case of basket crowns, the handle is thinned. Fitting of the crown consists of burnishing down the margins, checking the occlusion and cementing in place.

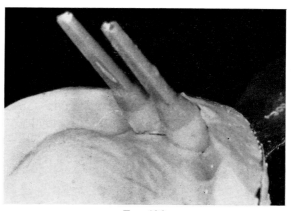

FIG. 106
Copper dies seated in transfer copings, prior to casting model.

Factors influencing Aesthetics

If too much tissue is removed from the incisal edge or proximal slices there will be an unsightly gold band along the edges of the tooth. The aim should be to maintain as much labial enamel as possible. All gold used in the front of the mouth should be contoured to avoid light reflection from a flat plane of gold.

Facings

If the area of tissue lost is large, acrylic or silicate facings may be placed. At the 'wax-up' stage, the area to be faced is carved

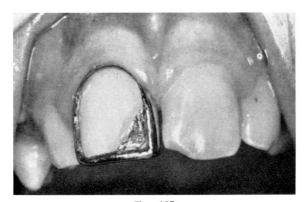

Fig. 107
Basket crown, prepared for facing.

out to form a box. When the casting is being finished, the box edges are further undercut with a small inverted cone bur to ensure retention for the facing material (Fig. 107). After cementing the crown, the box is filled with acrylic resin or silicate cement of a matching shade. It is possible to face the complete surface of a basket crown by slightly raising the gold margins to retain the facing material (Fig. 108).

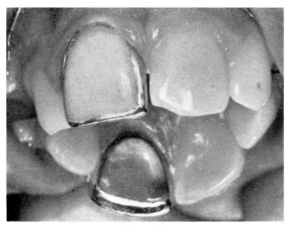

Fig. 108
Full labial facing of basket crown in acrylic.

NON-VITAL TEETH

If the tooth is non-vital and has received adequate root canal therapy, many of the objections to a permanent restoration at a younger age are eliminated.

The tooth which remains intact following injury occasionally becomes discoloured and may be treated by bleaching rather than crowning. Discoloration may appear almost immediately after injury as a result of rupture of pulpal vessels or subsequent pulpal death. Discoloration may also occur in injured teeth following root canal treatment.

Discoloured teeth are usually unsightly and, in a sensitive child, may create such an awareness that the offending tooth is persistently masked by the lip when talking or smiling. In most cases it is advisable to provide treatment which will improve the child's facial appearance. This can be done by removing the discoloured crown and fitting a post-core crown. An alternative method of treatment, and one worth considering in suitable cases, is to bleach the discoloured crown. This should only be undertaken as an interim measure to delay crowning for several years. In the latter procedure, careful selection of cases is important and the following criteria should be met:

1. The root filling must hermetically seal the apex of the tooth and the periapical tissues must be sound.
2. Small carious areas or small restorations are acceptable, but bleaching is contra-indicated in teeth which have extensive caries or large restorations.
3. The enamel must be free from cracks.

Bleaching for Permanent Anterior Teeth

Protection of the patient from the bleaching agent, 30 per cent hydrogen peroxide, is best provided by a large sheet of polythene sheeting. This provides overall coverage.

At the first visit:

1. Thoroughly clean the teeth with prophylactic paste.
2. Remove all caries and leaking fillings.
3. Open the pulp chamber widely, including the pulp horns. Remove the root filling to just below the gingival margin level. Remove any excess sealing agent with a mixture of equal parts of xylol and 95 per cent alcohol.
4. Before applying rubber dam apply a topical anaesthetic

and protect the contiguous soft tissue with petroleum jelly. Isolate only the affected tooth with rubber dam. Use a double floss silk ligature and maintain this in place with a butterfly clamp.

5. Cleanse all debris from the pulp chamber, canal and tooth surface with chlorinated soda B.P. followed by hydrogen peroxide, 10 vol.

6. Irrigate with warm water.

7. Dry the tooth and dehydrate all the tooth surfaces and pulp chamber with a mixture of one part ethyl alcohol and two parts chloroform.

8. Place a napkin over the patient's eyes. This will provide protection from the 30 per cent hydrogen peroxide and also from the photo-flood beam.

9. Use the bleaching agent, 30 per cent hydrogen peroxide, applied on wisps of cotton-wool to the pulp chamber and all surfaces of the tooth. A photo-flood beam is applied for 5 minutes whilst the cotton-wool wisps are kept moistened with the bleaching agent. This procedure is repeated four times.

10. Any cavities are then filled with oxyphosphate cement. A small pledget of cotton-wool dampened with the 30 per cent hydrogen peroxide is placed in the pulp chamber and this is sealed in position with oxyphosphate cement. The cement is held firmly in place until set with a piece of rubber dam lightly coated with petroleum jelly.

11. The rubber dam is removed and the improvement in colour noted. It is well to bear in mind that the isolation from moisture and the dehydration of the tooth alone can cause an appreciable lightening in colour of the tooth. A subsequent appointment is made in a week's time.

At the second visit:

Check the shade and if necessary bleach the tooth again, following the procedure of the first visit.

If the bleaching is successful a self-curing acrylic monomer is used to restore the translucency and to seal the dentinal tubules. It is applied to the pulp chamber and all tooth surfaces and exposed to the photo-flood beam for 5 minutes.

All cavities in the teeth can then be filled with a suitable shade of silicate filling material.

If the bleaching is unsuccessful after the two visits, it is advisable to abandon this form of treatment.

REFERENCE

BARRIE, W. J. M. & HARGREAVES, J. A. (1969). Stainless steel crowns in children's dentistry. *Dent. News, Lond.* **6**, No. 6, 8.

MARKLEY, M. R. (1958). Pin reinforcement and retention of amalgam foundations and restorations. *J. Am. dent. Ass.* **56**, 675.

CHAPTER 7

Total Displacement of a Tooth

WHEN a tooth is totally displaced through trauma or on those relatively rare occasions when a tooth is subsequently extracted, special consideration must be given to the planning of treatment in relation to the dentition as a whole, but emergency treatment appropriate to the situation must be carried out without delay.

Immediate treatment is confined to the remoulding of the socket, which can be corrected by gentle pressure between index finger and thumb, and to the treatment of any soft tissue injury. Attention should be paid to both adjacent and opposing teeth to eliminate the possibility of their involvement. Following immediate attention, the patient should be dismissed for at least 48 hours to permit soft tissue oedema to subside before a decision is taken on the best course of treatment to be followed. Unless the soft tissue injuries are severe, further treatment should not be delayed beyond this period. Failure to institute the correct treatment promptly may lead to complications much more difficult to treat subsequently since, in all cases where tooth loss has occurred, the teeth on either side of the space created will tilt towards it.

Consider further the possible consequences if no treatment is undertaken in a given situation.

Maxillary Loss

If the incisor relationship is normal and there is a good tooth/tissue relationship with no overcrowding, then tilting of the adjacent teeth and space closure will be minimal. In Angle Class I malocclusion, however, with a poor tooth/tissue relationship, closure of the space will occur rapidly and often completely.

If an incisor is lost in an Angle Class II malocclusion, where

the abnormal incisor relationship may be due to mesial movement of the buccal segments, closure of the space will be
accompanied by further forward drifting of the buccal segment,
particularly on the side of tooth loss, and will complicate an
already difficult orthodontic problem.

Loss of a maxillary incisor in an Angle Class III malocclusion
may increase the tendency to a lingual occlusion if left untreated.

Mandibular Loss

When loss occurs in the mandibular incisor region, both
the incisor relationship and the tooth/tissue ratio will again
influence what happens.   If the relationship is normal and
the tooth/tissue ratio favourable, tilting and closure will be
minimal.

If the relationship is Angle Class II, loss of a mandibular
incisor may lead to a lingual collapse of the lower anterior
segment and may also increase the severity of the existing
malocclusion.

If, however, the relationship is Angle Class III, lingual collapse of the mandibular anterior segment could lead to some
improvement in the malocclusion.   Loss of a mandibular incisor
may also affect the maxillary arch by inducing a secondary
collapse in that arch leading to imbrication of the maxillary
incisors.

In the assessment of Class V injuries, it is, therefore, clearly
important to take note of such factors as incisor relationship,
tooth/tissue ratio, and skeletal pattern so that treatment may
be planned to provide a good final result from the points of view
of both aesthetics and function.

Treatment

Loss of Maxillary Central Incisor.   When a maxillary incisor
is lost through injury two lines of treatment are possible.   The
space can either be maintained with a view to replacing the lost
tooth by a suitably designed prosthesis at the appropriate time
or the space may be allowed to close.   In the latter choice the
objective is to achieve the best possible position and axial
inclination of the lateral incisor in order to permit the placement
of an aesthetically pleasing jacket crown restoration.   This can
only be achieved satisfactorily by a fixed appliance so that

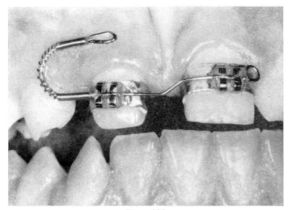

FIG. 109

Fixed appliance to move a maxillary lateral incisor mesially
into position of missing central incisor.

bodily movement of the tooth to the correct position is achieved
(Figs 109 and 110). The use of a removable appliance in these
cases should not be attempted since this will result in a tipping
movement of the tooth about its apex which will be aesthetically
unacceptable.

In cases of normal occlusion space maintenance would be the
treatment of choice. If the loss occurs early, at a time when the

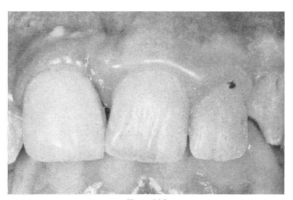

FIG. 110

Clinical photograph of realigned and crowned maxillary
lateral incisor tooth to simulate a central incisor.

H

abutment teeth are not fully developed, a removable space maintainer of the type shown in Figure 111 is indicated.

If the space is maintained in an Angle Class I or Angle Class II malocclusion the case will be treated as though no loss had occurred and this may entail extractions in the buccal segment

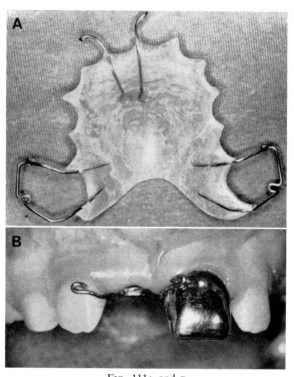

FIG. 111A and B

A removable space maintainer. A shows completed space maintainer; B shows space maintainer in position in the mouth.

at the appropriate time to provide space for the alignment of the anterior teeth. However, if the space created by the loss is used to align the incisor teeth, no further extraction may be necessary and the period of orthodontic treatment may be considerably reduced.

Should loss occur at an early age in Class I or Class II malocclusions and before preparation for a full porcelain crown is desirable, two lines of procedure are possible as soon as the lateral incisor is in the desired position. Firstly, a temporary crown may be fitted after minimal preparation of the immature tooth or, secondly, the lateral incisor may be held in the desired position either by a fixed or well-designed removable appliance until satisfactory crowning is feasible. The latter is the more satisfactory method. In such cases the final appearance is further improved by progressive stoning of the canine to simulate the lateral incisor (Fig. 112).

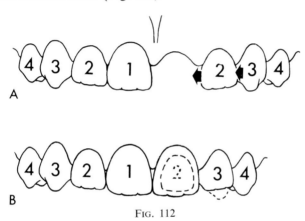

FIG. 112

Utilisation of space to realign maxillary incisor teeth.
A controlled closure following loss of a central incisor;
B restoration of acceptable appearance by crowning of the
lateral incisor and progressive stoning of the canine.

In Angle Class III cases, injury to the maxillary incisor teeth is a rare occurrence. Maintenance of the space is essential during early corrective orthodontic procedures, but no attempt should be made during this period to fit a prosthesis. After the initial stage of orthodontic treatment, a partial denture designed also to act as a space maintainer should be fitted.

Clearly the decision on which method of treatment to adopt is a matter of judgement and experience involving not only a knowledge of occlusal classification and skeletal pattern but also including a consideration of such other factors as the suitability of the lateral incisor for crowning and the importance to the patient of good dental appearance. Thus, the sex of the patient and the position of the lip line are additional factors which should be taken into account. Finally, it can be said that the treatment of each case requires to be planned on its individual merits.

Loss of Maxillary Lateral Incisor. Loss of a maxillary lateral incisor presents special problems, sometimes difficult to resolve satisfactorily. In cases with tooth/tissue imbalance and incisor imbrication, it is better to use the space created for realignment of the incisor teeth, except possibly in special cases where good dental appearance is essential when maintenance of space, followed by correction of the malocclusion and the placement of a prosthesis would be preferable.

When it is decided to use the space created for realignment of the anterior teeth it follows that this process must be controlled and not permitted to take place in a haphazard fashion. It is essential to establish the axial inclination of the unerupted canine teeth since this will provide a guide to the prognosis for an acceptable result. A distally inclined canine provides a favourable indication when a lateral incisor is lost, while a mesially inclined canine is a definite contra-indication.

Occasionally it happens that the lateral incisor on the opposite side of the same arch, where loss has occurred, is not of normal size and shape. In these circumstances it is often better to extract this tooth and allow both canines to move mesially. The final appearance will be improved when the tip of the canine tooth is progressively stoned to simulate a lateral incisor.

Loss of a Mandibular Central or Lateral Incisor. Since total displacement of an incisor tooth results from direct trauma, the loss of a mandibular incisor is a comparatively rare occurrence as this tooth is protected by the lower lip. Should a lower incisor be lost through trauma or extraction following the injury, controlled closure by means of a fixed appliance is necessary. In this way, collapse of the mandibular anterior segment and possible mal-alignment of the maxillary incisors may be avoided. While maintenance of the space would also achieve the same result, a satisfactory lower prosthesis is difficult to achieve and undesirable in itself.

Total Displacement of Deciduous Teeth

The premature loss of a deciduous incisor should never be regarded as trivial since, apart from the possible adverse dental effects, psychological trauma may result from the child being aware that he is different from others of the same age.

In general, the sequelae following loss of a deciduous incisor are similar to those for the permanent tooth.

Loss of a Maxillary or Mandibular Central Incisor. Loss of either a maxillary or mandibular central incisor in a well-spaced primary dentition indicating a favourable tooth/tissue ratio, will not result in closure of the space even if lost early, and no active treatment is required then or later. The child, however, should be kept under observation for the possible development of undesirable non-dental sequelae.

In the primary dentition which has an unfavourable tooth/ tissue ratio seen as lack of spacing or imbrication of the labial segment, particularly when loss occurs before the age of 4, closure of the space may follow. If the anterior crowding is due to mesial movement of the buccal segments Walther (1966) believes that closure of the space will be accompanied by further drifting of the buccal segments, thereby increasing the irregularity in the permanent dentition. Opinion differs on the need for space maintenance in such cases. Finn (1967) believes that an anterior space maintainer is indicated when loss occurs early or in a crowded primary dentition. However, since orthodontic treatment will invariably be required during the mixed dentition period, no useful purpose is served by initiating treatment at this early stage. Space maintenance is, therefore, not recommended in the primary dentition. The one exception occurs when multiple loss of primary teeth is involved. In such cases a partial denture, so designed that it does not interfere with inter-canine growth, will improve function and restore confidence (Hargreaves, 1964; Laird, 1966). Both Baume (1950) and Clinch (1951) have shown that little lateral growth of the jaws occurs between about $2\frac{1}{2}$ and 6 years of age. This is the period during which deciduous tooth extraction might have to be undertaken. A growth spurt occurs which is seen as an increase in inter-canine width at, or a little before, the eruption of the permanent incisors. It should be noted that in both the maxillary and the mandibular arches inter-canine growth is greater in the previously unspaced primary dentition than in the previously spaced primary dentition.

Loss of Maxillary or Mandibular Lateral Incisor. If the tooth lost is a maxillary or mandibular lateral incisor, in an unspaced primary dentition a swing of the midline will take place unless the loss is counterbalanced by the extraction of the other lateral in the same arch. Lingual collapse of the maxillary segment will be prevented by the intact lower arch. This extraction can be regarded as the first step in a process of serial extractions designed to provide adequate space for the permanent incisor teeth. Similarly, in an unspaced mandibular arch, loss of a lateral incisor should be counterbalanced by extraction of the other lateral in the same arch.

REFERENCES

BAUME, L. J. (1950). Physiological tooth migration and its significance for the development of occlusion. *J. dent. Res.* **29**, 123.

CLINCH, L. M. (1951). Analysis of serial models between three and eight years of age. *Dent. Rec.* **71**, 61.

FINN, S. B. (1967). *Clinical Pedodontics*, 3rd ed. Philadelphia: Saunders.

HARGREAVES, J. A. (1964). Deciduous dentures. *Dent. News, Lond.* **2**, No. 1, 1.

LAIRD, W. R. (1966). Dentures for children. *Br. dent. J.* **121**, 385.

WALTHER, D. P. (1966). *Current Orthodontics*. Bristol: Wright.

CHAPTER 8

Permanent Restorations

THE treatment of traumatic injuries to the anterior teeth of children is frequently incomplete until near adulthood, when finally the operator is primarily concerned with the patient's appearance.

In those cases of injury resulting in loss of tooth tissue or of vitality with subsequent discoloration of the crown, consideration must be given to the nature of the final restoration. It is, however, beyond the scope of this textbook to describe in detail the techniques for the various anterior restorations available but, in giving consideration to the appropriate treatment, certain guiding principles are worthy of note.

In the recently traumatised tooth the objectives of treatment are to place the injured tooth at rest, to maintain total arch length and to avoid further trauma to the young pulp which might arise from extensive preparation. There also exists the danger in an immature tooth of damage by traumatic exposure to the relatively large pulp. In addition, further eruption of the tooth during the developmental stages will expose any preparation of the gingival margin, making a new restoration mandatory to restore appearance. For these reasons permanent crowning of the anterior teeth is not advised before the age of 16 or 17 years.

ASSESSMENT OF PATIENT

Before proceeding to the final treatment it is always pertinent to assess the patient's attitude towards dental health. Teeth missing by extraction, untreated caries or the existence of poor oral hygiene, usually serve as contra-indications to advanced restorations. The patient's attitude towards the proposed treatment is also of some importance, since he may prove unwilling to co-operate in the successful completion of the restoration.

Clinical Assessment

A full clinical reassessment of the case is required at this stage and should include the following tests:

Vitality. Although the case notes may record that follow-up vitality tests have been made at regular intervals and that vitality has been maintained, this should be checked once more before proceeding to the final restoration.

Periodontal Condition. Any periodontal condition, even if confined to a local gingivitis, must be noted and treated before proceeding to the crown preparation since later treatment of a gingival condition will lead to some recession of the gingival margin and thus detract from the appearance of the final restoration (Fig. 113).

Axial Inclination of Tooth. In a previously untreated or inadequately treated injury some loss of mesio-distal space may have occurred as the result of mesial inclination or less frequently proclination of the involved tooth (Fig. 114). The mesially inclined tooth presents two problems. Firstly, the mesial pulp horn is at risk during the course of crown preparation, and secondly, it may be impossible to fit a copper ring for impression taking (Fig. 115). In such cases it is tempting to restore the lost tissue with a Class IV inlay, pin-inlay, gold foil, or pin-reinforced anterior filling material. Seldom do such restorations have a satisfactory appearance and consideration should be given to endodontic treatment followed by a post-core jacket crown.

Occlusion. The occlusion should be checked both in centric occlusion and in lateral excursions of the mandible since a heavy anterior bite will dictate the fitting of a crown suitably modified to withstand the occlusal stresses.

Radiographic Examination. Radiographic examination is required to complete the pre-operative assessment for the following reasons:

1. To establish the size and position of the pulp relative to the line of fracture;
2. To eliminate the possibility of periapical pathology;
3. To confirm the presence of a satisfactory root filling in a non-vital tooth;
4. To establish adequate root length for the provision of a post.

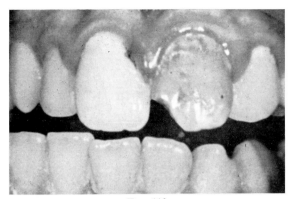

FIG. 113
Untreated gingival condition associated with traumatised
anterior teeth.

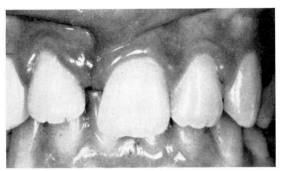

FIG. 114
Space loss associated with untreated traumatised anterior
teeth.

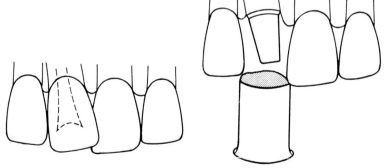

FIG. 115
Axial inclination of maxillary central incisor preventing
normal fitting of a copper ring (after Kantorowicz).

CHOICE OF RESTORATION

The choice of restoration depends almost solely on the clinical findings in each case, but the following crowns are all permissible restoration in a given situation.

Porcelain Jacket Crown. The porcelain jacket crown is a restoration of excellent appearance which is well tolerated by the soft tissues and, because of its low conductivity, protects the pulp from thermal shock. Although it has a low impact strength and tends to fracture easily, it has a Brinell hardness of 415 and therefore wears well. It is impervious to oral fluids and does not stain easily. The material is radio-opaque and may thus be readily identified on radiographs.

Aluminous porcelain is increasing in popularity as a material suitable for jacket crowns and may well, in time, replace conventional porcelain altogether. Its success is well founded on good appearance, high strength and greater resistance to torque due to its high modulus of elasticity. McLean (1967), in a review of 1,334 aluminous crowns over a period of three and a half years, confirms that these crowns withstand torque better than the conventional porcelains, and reports a fracture rate of less than 0·5 per cent.

Indications for Porcelain Jacket Crown. The indications for a porcelain jacket crown are as follows:

1. Class II fracture, vital pulp, where sufficient tooth tissue remains to provide adequate support.
2. Crowning of lateral incisor when previously moved into correct position and axial inclination by orthodontic procedures, to resemble central incisor.
3. Absence of heavy anterior bite.
4. Satisfactory radiographic evidence of sound periapical condition.
5. Absence of periodontal disease.
6. Good oral hygiene.
7. Interest in dental health, and adequate signs of willing co-operation.

Porcelain Bonded to Gold Crowns. In cases of heavy anterior bite the use of porcelain as a crown material is contra-indicated because of the liability of fracture. In such cases the crown is fabricated from gold, thus providing sufficient strength to withstand the biting stresses while the requirements of appearance are satisfied by a specially developed porcelain (Fig. 116).

Acrylic Jacket Crowns. While the acrylic crown is occasionally useful as a semi-permanent restoration it is not recommended as a permanent restoration, since it suffers from a number of serious disadvantages when compared with porcelain. Because its coefficient of thermal expansion is seven times higher than tooth substance, changes in mouth temperature break the cement seal and result in poor peripheral adaptation. Acrylic resin is comparatively soft and is susceptible to wear and discoloration. Further acrylic crowns are radiolucent and therefore difficult to detect if inhaled.

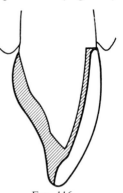

FIG. 116

Porcelain bonded to gold crown.

Since the life of an acrylic crown is limited periodic replacement is inevitable.

Shoulderless Crowns. The construction of a shoulderless crown as such is not advised since both porcelain and acrylic are weak in thin section. However, in a number of cases, such as the peg-shaped lateral incisor or the lower incisor, the preparation of a shoulder may endanger the pulp. In such cases the shoulder is provided as part of an open-ended cast-gold thimble fitted over the shoulderless preparation (Fig. 117).

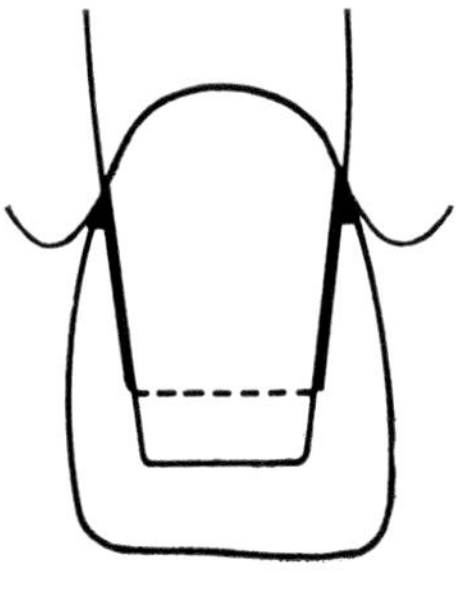

FIG. 117

Fabrication of a shoulder with an open-ended cast gold thimble fitted to a shoulderless preparation (after Kantorowicz).

Cast Core Post Crown. If root canal therapy is necessary as, for example, in a pulp previously treated by pulpotomy or if a root filling is already present, the tooth will be weakened by the access opening and by the brittle nature of the devitalised dentine. The position may be further complicated by the degree of loss of tooth tissue resulting from trauma or by malalignment of the tooth. Such teeth are best treated by a cast core post crown (Fig. 118).

Indications for Cast Core Post Crown. The indications for a cast core post crown are as follows:

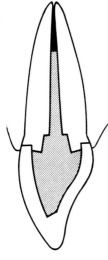

1. Class III fracture or Class II fracture previously treated as Class III.
2. Rotated or malaligned teeth.
3. Discoloured teeth.
4. No periapical pathology.
5. Satisfactory apical-third root filling.
6. Adequate root length to support crown.
7. Absence of local or general periodontal condition.
8. Good oral hygiene.
9. Satisfactory attitude of patient to dental health and adequate signs of willing co-operation.

FIG. 118

Cast core post crown.

The Malaligned Tooth

Reference has been made earlier to the difficulties involved in preparation and impression taking for the malaligned vital tooth. In the case of the pulpless tooth it is possible, within limits, to realign a mesially inclined crown by altering the angle of the core relative to the line of the post. In cases of heavy anterior bite a slight realignment of the axial inclination of the core labially will serve to clear the bite, thus obviating the need for a gold palatal surface.

Other Restorative Methods

A number of other methods including gold and porcelain inlays, pinlays, gold foil, acrylic and silicate cements reinforced with stainless-steel pins are feasible but all such methods are less satisfactory as permanent restorations and frequently more hazardous than the appropriate full crown as outlined above.

REFERENCES

McLean, J. W. (1967). The alumina reinforced porcelain jacket crown. *J. Am. dent. Ass.* **75**, 621.

FURTHER READING

Chapman, C. E. (1969). *Manual of Dental Operative Technique.* Edinburgh: Livingstone.
Kantorowicz, G. F. (1963). *Inlays, Crowns and Bridges. A Clinical Handbook.* Bristol: Wright.

CHAPTER 9

Injuries to Deciduous Teeth

A SURVEY by Schreiber (1959) of 118 children who received trauma to their deciduous teeth showed most of these children suffered this injury between $1\frac{1}{2}$ and $2\frac{1}{2}$ years of age.

This is the time in a child's development when his walking and running activities become adventurous, making him subject to repeated tumbles. It is also the time when developmentally the roots of the anterior teeth are fully formed with maximum anchorage, a fact which influences both the type of injury sustained and the subsequent treatment possible.

The injuries to deciduous teeth can be classified in a similar way to that already described for permanent teeth.

Partial Displacement by Direct Trauma

If the blow is direct, the displacement follows one of three movements:

1. A palatal or lingual movement with fracture of the palatal or lingual alveolar bone (Fig. 119A).
2. A palatal or lingual movement with fracture of the labial alveolar bone (Fig. 119B).
3. Displacement of the tooth from its socket, the tooth appears elongated on clinical examination (Fig. 119C).

Partial Displacement by Indirect Trauma

In these cases, the time of injury is very critical if tooth intrusion occurs, since development of the permanent successor could be affected depending on the amount of its crown formation.

The displacement again follows one of three movements:

1. A labial movement with fracture of the palatal or lingual alveolar bone and compression of the labial alveolar bone (Fig. 119D).

2. A labial movement with fracture of the labial alveolar
   bone (Fig. 119E).
3. Intrusion of the tooth into its socket compressing bone
   in the periapical region, the tooth appearing short or in
   some cases completely intruded into the alveolar bone
   (Fig. 119F and G).

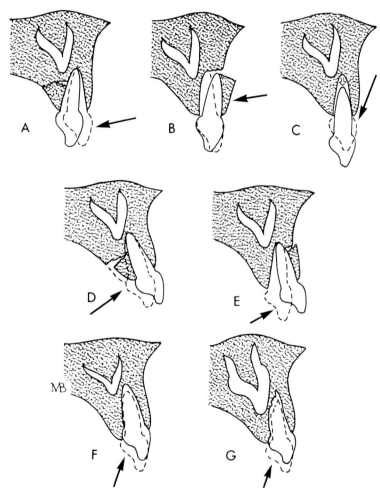

FIG. 119A–G

Types of tooth displacement following direct and indirect trauma.

Total Displacement due to Trauma

Complete loss of a deciduous tooth can occur. The cause of such displacement is usually due to direct trauma. As the deciduous tooth approaches its normal time for shedding, the resorption of the root will be so advanced that total displacement can easily result from a direct blow at this age.

Fracture due to Trauma

Fracture of anterior deciduous teeth is less common than displacement, in contrast to injuries of the permanent teeth. This is due to the thinner compact bone in young children. The labial plate is very thin, and the underlying cancellous bone is loosely trabeculated.

The deciduous anterior teeth are placed in a more vertical position in the alveolar bone when they are compared with permanent teeth and this may encourage tooth displacement rather than fracture.

In cases of indirect trauma, intrusion may be facilitated by passage into the underlying crypt of a permanent tooth (Fig. 119F and G).

When fracture of a deciduous tooth does occur, it can be typed in the same way as permanent teeth.

Type I   Simple fracture of the crown not involving dentine.

Type II   Extensive fracture of the crown involving both enamel and dentine but not exposing the dental pulp.

Type III   Extensive fracture of the crown exposing the dental pulp.

Type IV   Fracture of the root with or without coronal fracture.

Assessment of Injury with Aims and Principles of Treatment

The assessment of injury may be difficult in a very young child who is frightened and shocked following his accident. Miller (1962) describes an excellent method for examining babies and very young children. Visual access to the mouth can be obtained if the mother is seated on an ordinary chair with the child on her lap. The child's legs can be placed under the mother's arm. The operator seated opposite the mother receives the child's head into his lap, the mother holding the child's hands with her own (Fig. 120).

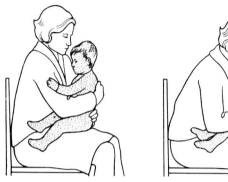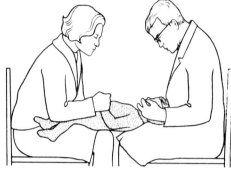

FIG. 120
Oral examination of a small child.

If the child should be restless, the operator can support the child's head with his wrists, and visual examination and mouth access is easily facilitated.   Both upper and lower arches can be seen and if there is the possibility of a finger being bitten, the index finger held behind the deciduous molars will prevent the child closing heavily during the examination.

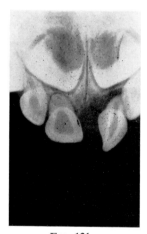

FIG. 121
Radiograph following maxillary injury in a young child,
showing displacement of
maxillary incisors.

After taking a history, palpation of the teeth can be completed by the method previously described in Chapter 2.

Radiographs are difficult in some cases, but adequate examination of the anterior segments can be obtained by using a periapical radiograph in an occlusal position (Fig. 121), the child holding the film between the teeth rather than supporting the film by hand.

Pulp testing by any of the conventional methods is not advisable as the response from a very young child cannot be relied upon.

Treatment

The emergency treatment must take into account both general and local injury and infection. If the patient is in a general state of clinical shock or has suffered severe injury, he should be treated for this immediately and returned to his home or hospital under medical supervision. In these circumstances the local treatment of the injured teeth is temporarily delayed. As previously discussed, consideration of the place of injury must be made in respect of possible tetanus infection and preventive methods against tetanus given as soon as possible. At the first

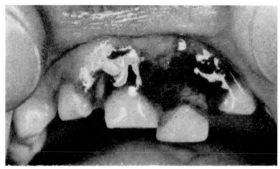

Fig. 122

Recent injury to deciduous teeth, illustrating apparent extensive haemorrhage and soft tissue involvement.

examination following the injury, treatment for any soft tissue involvement must be assessed and adequate control instigated. The same procedures for treatment of soft tissue damage outlined in Chapter 4 should be followed.

The injury to a young child can be very alarming to the mother. A little blood mixed with saliva can give the impression of copious haemorrhage and clotting of blood on the lips can suggest extensive laceration (Fig. 122).

The initial examination should be short but thorough. The child can be examined in the manner outlined above, seated on the mother's lap.

The extent of the damage should be noted, but unless extensive laceration has occurred needing hospitalisation, or unless the teeth involved are badly fractured or displaced, nothing more than first aid care should be commenced.

I

First-Aid Care. The child is usually frightened or tearful soon after a facial injury. The first-aid care must aim at establishing adequate oral hygiene for the child. The face and mouth can be gently cleaned with a warm 2 per cent solution of sodium bicarbonate. The mother should be reassured if no extensive injury has been found. If the injury is severe, hospitalisation should be undertaken. The parent should be advised on home oral hygiene methods. This is best continued by gentle bathing of the affected area with warm 2 per cent sodium bicarbonate mouthwashes or swabbing of the affected area with cotton-wool soaked in the bicarbonate solution. Analgesics are advisable for one or two days following the injury.

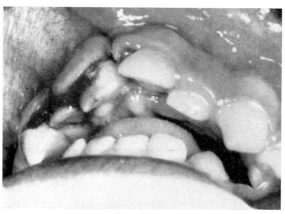

Fig. 123
Intrusion of maxillary anterior deciduous teeth.

The child's condition should then be reviewed in approximately 7 days' time. If the teeth are badly fractured with pulpal exposure, or are so loose that inhalation might occur, then extraction of those teeth should be undertaken under general anaesthetic, as soon as possible. Splinting of loose deciduous teeth or pulpotomy for fractured teeth with pulpal involvement is possible in a similar way to that described for permanent teeth, but for a very young child where co-operation is often difficult, radical treatment by extraction is the kindest course of treatment.

Fortunately tooth fracture is rare. Much more frequently,

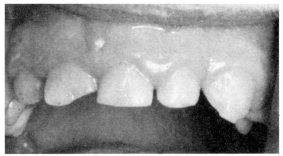

FIG. 124

Re-eruption of maxillary anterior teeth following intrusion.

however, a tooth can be intruded into the underlying bone and as long as this is not interfering with the occlusion is best left undisturbed. In many cases the tooth will re-erupt back into the arch and in some cases will remain vital (Figs 123 and 124). If the tooth does become non-vital, pulp therapy can be undertaken at a later date, when the child has recovered from the accident. Pulp treatment for non-vital deciduous anterior teeth can be completed in a similar way to the description in Chapter 5 for non-vital permanent teeth with open apices, but because of possible involvement by infection of the underlying developing permanent successional tooth, the first sign of pulpal death by crown discoloration or sinus formation is best treated by extraction.

Root fracture can occur (Fig. 125), but is also rare. Again, because of possible infection of the underlying developing

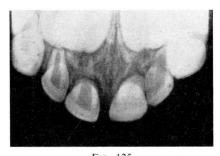

FIG. 125

Radiograph of root fracture of a maxillary
right deciduous incisor tooth.

permanent successional tooth, extraction of the fractured deciduous incisor including the apical fragment should be undertaken.

Follow-up Care. After first-aid treatment, the child should be seen again in about one week's time.

Chipped enamel edges can be smoothed by gently grinding with a sandpaper disc in a handpiece. More extensive crown fractures with no pulpal involvement can be capped with stainless-steel deciduous crowns in a similar way to that already described for permanent teeth (Fig. 126), but unless full co-

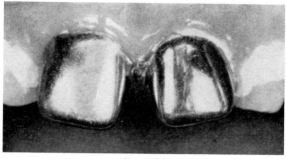

Fig. 126

Stainless steel crowns protecting maxillary deciduous incisor teeth.

operation of the child is achieved, this treatment is best delayed and the tooth kept under observation. If no symptoms occur, the tooth can be left until its normal shedding time but if it gives rise to pain or becomes non-vital it should be extracted.

Displaced teeth should be kept under continuous review. If they give rise to pain or become non-vital, they are better removed. As already described, many intruded teeth gradually re-erupt over a one- to six-month period. In such cases no treatment other than observation and reassurance to the mother is required, provided that they re-erupt with no occlusal interference.

A further clinical examination with radiographs should be taken six months after the injury and any periapical pathology found at this time should be treated by immediate extraction. It cannot be stressed too strongly that possible infection of the

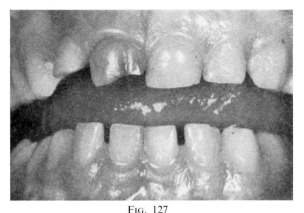

FIG. 127
Discoloured non-vital maxillary deciduous central incisor.

developing permanent successional teeth should be eliminated by extraction of a non-vital deciduous predecessor.

A child suffering injury to a deciduous tooth should have regular six-monthly examinations following the initial treatment until the tooth is shed and the permanent successor is in place.

Sequelae to Injuries of Deciduous Teeth

The most common result of injury to a deciduous tooth is pulpal death followed by discoloration (Fig. 127). Periapical infection can result from pulpal death which is usually shown clinically by a sinus (Fig. 128) or radiographically as a

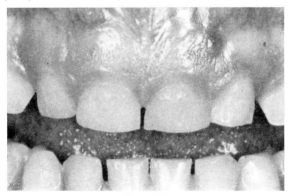

FIG. 128
Sinus development following pulpal death of a maxillary deciduous central incisor.

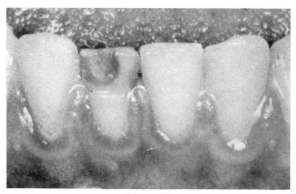

FIG. 129

Hypoplastic mandibular right permanent central incisor.

radiolucent area at the tooth apex. Very rarely does a radicular cyst form in the short period of time following pulp death and normal exfoliation of that tooth.

Injury to the underlying permanent successional tooth can occur. Schreiber (1959), who followed 118 patients found that eight permanent teeth had some sign of the injury.

The injury to the permanent successor will depend on the developmental age of the child when the accident occurred. Rushton (1956, 1958), Schreiber (1959) and Ball (1965) have described some of these sequelae which include dilaceration, hypoplastic enamel, partial duplication and aberrant calcification.

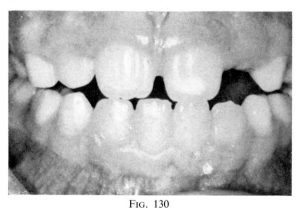

FIG. 130

Hypocalcific spots in maxillary permanent left central incisor.

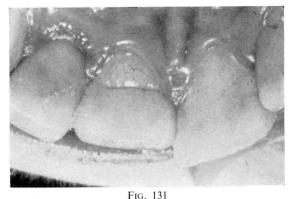

FIG. 131

Dilaceration of a maxillary permanent central incisor crown.

The most common sequelae are hypoplastic lesions (Turner teeth) where part of the crown has failed to develop normally (Fig. 129). Hypocalcific spots (white trauma spots) can be seen in areas of abnormal mineralisation of the crown of the successional permanent tooth (Fig. 130).

Severe trauma can result in dilaceration of crown or root (Fig. 131) of the permanent tooth, or in some cases total arrest of development, but this is very rare.

Occasionally the injured deciduous tooth will fail to resorb in the normal way (Fig. 132) and can result in the ectopic eruption of the permanent successor (Fig. 133).

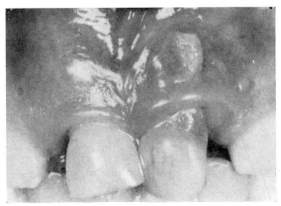

FIG. 132

Non-resorption of root; maxillary deciduous central incisor.

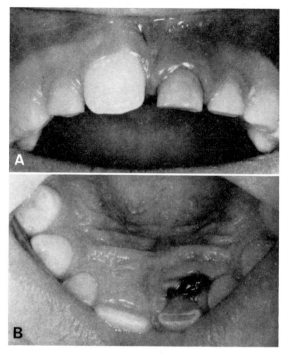

Fig. 133A and B
Palatal eruption of a maxillary permanent central incisor.

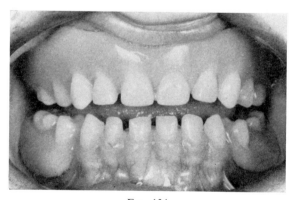

Fig. 134
Full upper and partial lower denture replacing teeth for a
4-year-old child.

The defects of tooth formation or abnormal path of eruption are due either to the severity of the force of the injury or to sepsis following pulpal death of the traumatised deciduous tooth.

Total Loss or Extraction of Anterior Deciduous Teeth

Loss of a deciduous anterior tooth is fully discussed in Chapter 7. In general it may be said that while the sequence of events is similar to that of loss of a permanent tooth, space maintenance is seldom required but for reasons of function and appearance, partial dentures may be desirable (Fig. 134).

REFERENCES

BALL, J. S. (1965). A sequel to trauma involving the deciduous incisors. *Br. dent. J.* **118**, 394.

MILLER, J. (1962). Dentistry for children. Acute conditions and problems of diagnosis. *Br. dent. J.* **112**, 182.

RUSHTON, M. A. (1956). Some late results of injury to teeth. *Br. dent. J.* **100**, 299.

RUSHTON, M. A. (1958). Partial duplication following injury to developing incisors. *Br. dent. J.* **104**, 9.

SCHREIBER, C. K. (1959). The effect of trauma on the anterior deciduous teeth. *Br. dent. J.* **106**, 340.

CHAPTER 10

The Prevention of Injuries

THE concept of preventive medicine has long been acknowledged and accepted as making an invaluable contribution to national health but preventive dentistry has made only slow progress to date. Even today preventive dentistry is only beginning to receive its rightful place on the dental curriculum and its acceptance by the public at large remains extremely limited. Such acceptance as does exist remains largely in the area of caries prevention and to a lesser extent in the prevention of periodontal diseases. The concept of interceptive orthodontics and the prevention of dental accidents continues to remain almost wholly in the province of the dental surgeon.

While traumatic injuries to the anterior teeth of children may occur in a variety of ways, changing leisure activities, including wider participation in sport of all kinds and the ever-increasing use of the motor car as a means of transport, will undoubtedly increase the risk. The incidence of such injuries is already too high and must give cause for concern.

Children with Angle Class II Division I malocclusions and those with inadequate lip coverage are particularly at risk. Such children should be given advice early on how injuries occur and thus how they may be avoided. From the accident point of view Class II Division I malocclusions should be treated as early as possible to diminish the risk of accidental injury. With all malocclusions, however, there exists an optimum age for the speediest reduction of the malocclusion. In the case of the Angle Class II Division I malocclusion, this is best left until 10 or 11 years of age. Thus, below this age and during the period of orthodontic treatment, children with proclinated incisors should be advised to wear a mouth protector when engaged in contact sports or during the sporting activities of skiing, canoeing and trampolining which are increasing in popularity.

Construction of Mouth Protectors

Mouth protectors can be divided into three groups:

1. The manufactured type which has a space left into which a soft lining material is placed. The protector is then used as an impression tray and held in place until the lining material has set. The periphery can then be trimmed with a pair of scissors.
2. The thermoplastic type which is also obtained in manufactured form. This type is softened in hot water then moulded in the mouth whilst still plastic.
3. The individually or custom-made protector, which is constructed on a model of the patient's mouth. This type of protector is most frequently made from latex rubber, silicone rubber or poly-vinyl chloride.

Groups 1 and 2 above have certain advantages in that they are quickly fabricated at the chairside and may be quickly replaced. However, they have the disadvantages that in the first type, the soft lining material tends to harden and separate from the outer part, while the fit of both the first and second types is less than satisfactory.

The ideal properties of the mouth protector may be listed as follows:

1. The appliance should fit well.
2. The protector should extend as far as possible into the sulcus and provide protection for the supporting tissue as well as the teeth. It follows that a good impression should define all muscle attachments clearly.
3. The rubber should be thick enough in the anterior region to absorb any impact and to prevent the teeth injuring the lips.
4. When the teeth are in occlusion the tips of the lower anteriors should be covered.
5. There should be sufficient thickness of material to prevent the posterior teeth coming into contact.
6. Palatally the protector should be kept as thin as possible consistent with strength, so that it will not interfere with speech or breathing.

The only appliance which fulfils these requirements is the custom-made protector constructed on an accurate model.

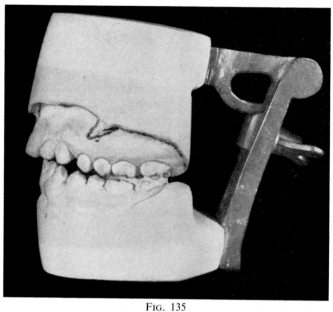

FIG. 135

Articulated models with the outline of the protector pencilled on the model and bite opened approximately 3 to 4 mm.

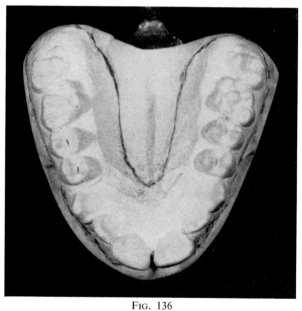

FIG. 136

Palatal aspect of the maxillary model, illustrating the extent of the palatal coverage.

Construction Technique for Latex Rubber Protector

The models are mounted in centric occlusion on a plane line articulator. The outline of the protector is pencilled on the model (Figs 135 and 136). The model is then given a coating of French chalk. A layer of modelling wax is laid down and cut to the pencilled outline. The bite is then opened 3 to 4 mm. and the wax built up until it contacts the lower teeth (Fig. 137). Labially the wax is also built out until the required thickness is obtained.

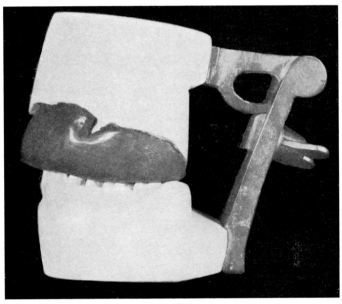

FIG. 137
Waxed up protector on articulator.

The thickness required is largely a matter of experience; it must not, however, be so thick that it cannot fit comfortably under the upper lip. The approximate thickness of wax over the different surfaces of the protector is illustrated in Figure 138A and B. The wax is smoothed and the periphery rounded off. The waxing up is finished by the addition of a thick round wax rod attached to the protector at each of the tuberosities (Fig. 139).

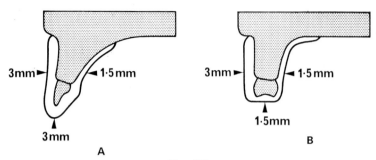

FIG. 138

Approximate thickness of wax in millimetres, over the different surfaces to be protected.

Plaster of Paris is mixed in a rubber bowl and vibrated to remove any air bubbles. The protector is then immersed on its model in the rubber bowl leaving the two wax rods protruding. When the plaster has set, it is removed from the bowl and placed in hot water. The wax is then boiled out and the mould left to cool.

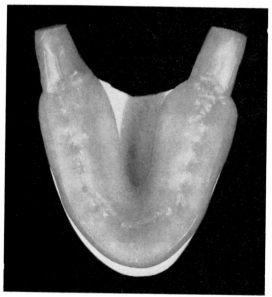

FIG. 139

Wax rods attached to the protector at each end of the tuberosities.

Gentle vibration is recommended while the latex is being poured. It should be noted that the latex rubber pours more easily when the mould is still damp. Latex shrinks during polymerisation and although this is not excessive with modern latex rubbers, the mould should be topped up at frequent intervals. To ensure that polymerisation shrinkage has been completed, 36 to 48 hours should elapse before removing the plaster.

The feed channels on the tuberosities are then cut off with a sharp scalpel or pair of scissors and a thin layer of latex smoothed over the attachment areas.

Finally the protector is placed on the master model to check the fit.

Instructions to Patient

The patient should be instructed to wash the protector free of saliva after use. This prevents the growth of bacteria and also prevents any deterioration in quality, if latex rubber has been used.

Conclusion

Since traumatic injuries are not confined to one group, consideration must be given to extending advice to all children at risk. It is the writers' belief that the prevention of dental accidents is too often a neglected area of advice and that the wider use of mouth protectors makes sound common sense.

Appendix of Laboratory Techniques

APPENDIX A

Acrylic Splint (Orthocryl Method)

Horsnell and Brown (1956) have described a rapid method of producing splints. The method detailed below describes a method for preparing a splint in Orthocryl which is rapid and effective (Orthocryl is a Dentauram product sold through Hawley, Russell and Baker Ltd., Potters Bar, Herts., England). The models are cast in a 50/50 plaster, Kaffir D mixture and trimmed. Any undercuts on the teeth are blocked out with plaster. The gingival margin is lightly scribed to ensure that the full coronal length of the tooth is utilised.

A thin retaining ridge of wax is built up round the gingival margins of the teeth. This will help to control the flow of Orthocryl while the splint is being constructed.

If the model is dry it is then necessary to soak in lukewarm water for approximately fifteen minutes, but a model already wet from the model trimmer requires only 5 minutes soaking. No separating medium is required when the model has been soaked.

A little Orthocryl powder is sprayed on to the model followed by just sufficient liquid to hold it in place. This technique is continued until the splint is completely built up. It is important that the liquid be applied sparingly since too much liquid will only result in the mix becoming too mobile to control.

The model is then immediately placed in a hydroflask. The water temperature should be 30 to 35°C and a pressure of 2·2 kg./cm.^{2} (30 lb per sq. in.) maintained for approximately 15 minutes.

Finally the model is removed and the splint trimmed and polished in the usual manner.

REFERENCE

HORSNELL, A. M. & BROWN, G. (1956). Immediate splints for cases of trauma to the incisor teeth. *Dent. Practnr. dent. Rec.* **6**, 148.

APPENDIX B

Cast Silver Fixed Splint

Remove any undercuts on the teeth by blocking out with plaster of Paris. Scribe round the gingival margins of the teeth to remove any imperfections. This will also ensure that the full coronal length of the tooth is being employed. Outline the design of the splint on the model. Apply french chalk, then

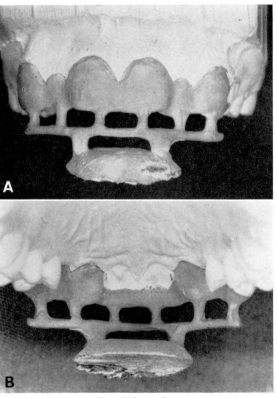

FIG. 140A and B

Cast silver splint showing the position of sprues; A from the labial aspect; B from the palatal aspect.

soften and adapt a sheet of gauge 8 (0·55) mm. casting wax. The adaption of the wax will be made much easier if a piece of cotton wool soaked in hot water is used. The wax is trimmed to the outline using a warm carver. Wax sprues, 2 mm. thick are directly inserted into the incisal edge of each tooth covered by the pattern and a 2 mm. wax rod unites each sprue. This spruing technique gives very satisfactory casting results (Fig. 140). The pattern is removed, coated with a suitable wetting agent and invested using Kerr's Cristobalite (Kerr, Europe S.p.A., Scafati (SA), Italy). It is then cast (Fig. 140) in casting silver (Ash 'Silver Casting Ingots' for splint work—Claudius Ash Sons and Co. Ltd., London, England). The sprues are removed with a cutting disc or fretsaw (not with cutting pliers), and the splint is polished.

Reverse Retention Gold Crown

Cast the model, remove the die and trim to the prepared margins, ensuring that the contact areas are a true representation of the tooth contour.

Lubricate both the die and the contact areas of the model with a suitable lubricant, for example, Kerr's microfilm (Kerr, Europe S.p.A., Scafati (SA), Italy). If a copper die is to be used, heat the die slightly in hot water before applying the lubricant to prevent chilling of the wax due to the thermal conductivity of the copper.

Apply a very thin layer of low-fusing inlay wax all over the die surface (for example Ruscher's Gusswachs, Erwin Ruscher, Zürich 2). This will facilitate removal of the crown and permit burnishing of the edges.

Replace the die in the model. Cut a piece of gauge 6 casting wax slightly longer and broader than the space to be filled;

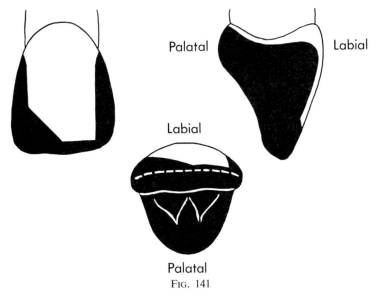

Palatal   Labial

Labial

Palatal

Fig. 141

Diagram to show fabrication of a reverse retention crown.

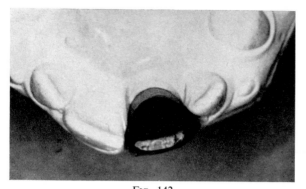

Fig. 142

Completed reverse retention crown in wax illustrating the
curvature of the incisal edge.

soften and adapt to the lingual surface of the die. Fill in the
mesial and the distal contact areas with blue inlay wax (Kerr
Regular Type II); add wax in small amounts to minimise the
danger of volumetric shrinkage and avoid over-heating the
wax; contour the lingual aspect and ensure that the reverse
retention areas are thick enough to resist distortion (Fig. 141).
Remove excess wax and trim to final outline, contouring the
incisal edge to the natural curve of the arch (Fig. 142). This is
important for both function and appearance. Smooth the
waxed up crown with a piece of nylon (for example nylon shirt
material) to eliminate the need for flaming.

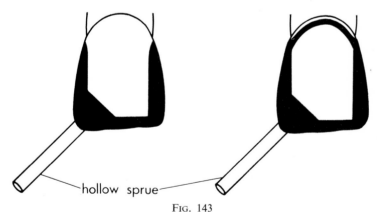

Fig. 143

Position of sprue for reverse retention and basket crowns.

Sprue from the mesial incisal corner at an angle of 45°
to the incisal edge (Fig. 143).   For centrifugal casting use a 2
mm. hollow sprue; for pressure casting use a 1·5 mm. sprue to
avoid the danger of a gravity cast.

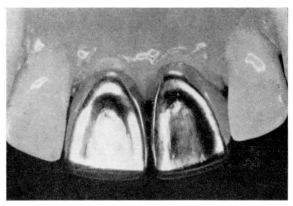

Fig. 144

Polished palatal surfaces of semi-permanent crowns, illustrating
polished contouring.

Finally the crown is invested, cast in gold and polished
(Fig. 144).   Kerr's Cristobalite is suggested as a suitable
investment material.   The gold advised is Cinormat (Johnson,
Matthey and Co. Ltd., Hatton Garden, London), a hard inlay
gold.

Basket Crown

The technique is basically the same as that for the reverse retention crown described in Appendix C. It differs only in the method of waxing the 'basket handle' and in obtaining an undercut area for the retention of the facing (Fig. 145).

The basket handle is formed by continuing the shoulders into the contour of the gingival margin in such a way that when the crown is fitted most of the handle will be concealed by the free gingiva. However, care should be taken to ensure that the wax is not carried into an undercut area beyond the preparation. The handle should be thick enough to resist distortion particularly at the points of union to the crown. Sufficient thickness of wax at these points also facilitates casting.

The margins bordering on the incisal, mesial and distal walls

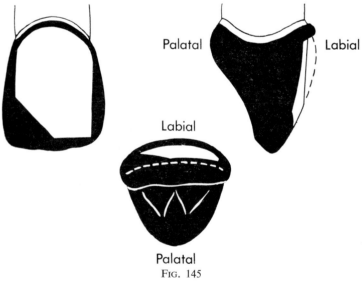

Palatal   Labial

Labial

Palatal

Fig. 145

Diagram to show fabrication of a basket crown.

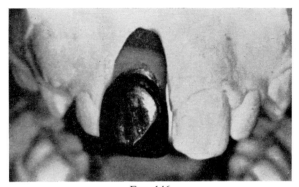

FIG. 146

Completed basket crown in wax, prior to casting,
prepared to receive a full facing.

of the labial surface should be undercut at the wax stage to
provide retention for a full or partial facing (Fig. 146).

The crown is sprued and finished in the same manner as the
reverse retention crown (Fig. 143).

Index

PRINTED BY T. & A. CONSTABLE LTD., EDINBURGH